Immunotoxicology

A Current Perspective of Principles and Practice

NATO ASI Series

Advanced Science Institutes Series

A series presenting the results of activities sponsored by the NATO Science Committee, which aims at the dissemination of advanced scientific and technological knowledge, with a view to strengthening links between scientific communities.

The Series is published by an international board of publishers in conjunction with the NATO Scientific Affairs Division

A Life Sciences **B Physics**	Plenum Publishing Corporation London and New York
C Mathematical and Physical Sciences	D. Reidel Publishing Company Dordrecht, Boston and Lancaster
D Behavioural and Social Sciences **E Applied Sciences**	Martinus Nijhoff Publishers Boston, The Hague, Dordrecht and Lancaster
F Computer and Systems Sciences **G Ecological Sciences**	Springer-Verlag Berlin Heidelberg New York Tokyo

Series G: Ecological Sciences No. 2

Immunotoxicology

A Current Perspective of Principles and Practice

Edited by

Peter W. Mullen

Kemic Bioresearch Laboratories Limited
P.O. Box 878, Kentville, Nova Scotia, Canada, B4N 4H8

Springer-Verlag Berlin Heidelberg New York Tokyo 1984
Published in cooperation with NATO Scientific Affairs Division

Proceedings of the NATO Advanced Study Institute on Immunotoxicology held at Acadia University, Wolfville, Nova Scotia, Canada, 14–23 July 1982

ISBN 3-540-13382-8 Springer-Verlag Berlin Heidelberg New York Tokyo
ISBN 0-387-13382-8 Springer-Verlag New York Heidelberg Berlin Tokyo

Printed in Germany

Printing: Beltz Offsetdruck, Hemsbach; Bookbinding: J. Schäffer OHG, Grünstadt
2131/3140-543210

ACKNOWLEDGEMENTS

In addition to the scientifically distinguished contributing authors, the editor is indebted to a number of people who assisted in the collation, retyping and proofreading of the papers contained in this text. Particular appreciation must be extended to both my technician, Elizabeth Ann McInnis, B.Sc. and to my dear wife, Susan, for their unfailing assistance and support.

P.W.M.

TABLE OF CONTENTS

IMMUNOTOXICOLOGY: BRIDGING A DISCIPLINE OR TWO

P.W. Mullen
Kemic Bioresearch Laboratories Limited
P.O. Box 878, Kentville, Nova Scotia
Canada, B4N 4H8

Attending the NATO Advanced Study Institute on Immunotoxicology on which this text is based, were physicians and scientists, both young and not so young, from seven countries. Biomedical scientists representing many different educational backgrounds including; immunologists, toxicologists, pharmacologists, pharmacists, biochemists, pathologists, general practitioners and basic biologists participated in the ten day meeting. Such a diversity of nationalities and talents indicates the ever growing interest in, and emphasizes a key characteristic of, immunotoxicology — namely, its interdisciplinary foundation and appeal.

In recent years, developments in immunopharmacology have provided ample evidence that a great range of therapeutic agents have the capacity to modulate immune responses. It should not be surprising therefore, that immunotoxicology, a natural offshoot of immunopharmacology, has now attracted the attention of biomedical researchers worldwide. Numerous reports have served to heighten the realization that many xenobiotics (chemicals 'foreign' to the body) may effect immunological changes, and both government regulatory agencies and industry have established divisions or departments of immunotoxicology in recent years. Of particular concern are the long-term and insidious immunological effects resulting from chronic exposure to low doses of various structurally unrelated compounds including drugs, food additives and those environmental pollutants as diverse as lead and 2,3,7,8-tetrachlorodibenzoparadioxin.

Like immunopharmacology (Mullen, 1979), immunotoxicology, and, for that matter, perhaps every fledgling interdisciplinary science, has progressed despite a lack of precise definition and clear objectives. Simply stated, immunotoxicology is the study of the adverse effects of xenobiotics on the body's immune system. Although seemingly clearcut according to this definition, to an external observer, it might appear that scientists working in this field fall into one of two main "camps" depending upon their training and research interests. These two groups, I shall label the "IMMUNOtoxicologists" and the "ImmunoTOXICOLOGISTS".

NATO ASI Series, Vol. G2
Immunotoxicology. Edited by P. W. Mullen

IMMUNOtoxicologists are by far the more numerous, and represent those researchers whose basic training was primarily in the area of immunology. Perhaps more "cell orientated" or "biological" in their approach, the IMMUNOtoxicologists, with their limited understanding of physico-chemical and pharmacological principles tend to perceive and interpret all immunotoxicological findings in terms of changes to the myriad "cell subpopulations" comprising the immune system. Often the IMMUNOtoxicologist will invoke the presence,and stress possible changes in the concentration,of a particular elusive "cell factor" or genuine lymphokine to facilitate an explanation of his or her findings.

Most ImmunoTOXICOLOGISTS on the other hand, received their basic education in pharmacology, toxicology or biochemistry. Consequently, the immunoTOXICOLOGIST may demonstrate a greater understanding of the importance of pharmacokinetics and biotransformation and considers the physico-chemical properties (e.g. pKa, lipid solubility, structure-activity relationship) of the xenobiotic *per se* when designing, or drawing conclusions from, each experiment.

Obviously, the advancement of our understanding of precisely how each xenobiotic affects the body's immune system will be dependent upon the findings and originality of both IMMUNOtoxicologists and immuno-TOXICOLOGISTS. Although somewhat biased, it is the author's opinion that the importance of pharmacokinetics and biotransformation, etc. should receive greater attention in the conduct of immunotoxicological research. A review of the scientific literature reveals that the results of many IMMUNOtoxicological investigations, particularly those conducted *in vitro*, could be re-interpreted by merely giving consideration to such basic pharmacological tenets as the "pH-partition hypothesis" and the consequences of binding to serum proteins (including fetal calf serum added *in vitro*) on xenobiotic activity. Only by utilizing to the fullest extent the techniques and theory of both the parent disciplines, immunology and toxicology, will the synthesis of a true immunotoxicology be achieved.

The NATO Advanced Study Institute afforded a unique opportunity to define and update the science of immunotoxicology through presentations of essential theory and relevant experimental findings by experts in various fields. The ASI meeting and this text will be deemed a success if the demarcation between IMMUNOtoxicology and ImmunoTOXICOLOGY is rendered less evident and the reader gains a better insight into the true interdisciplinary nature of this important branch of toxicological research.

REFERENCE

MULLEN, P.W. (1979) An immunopharmacology journal: Reflections on its interdisciplinary and historical context. Int J. Immunopharmac. 1, 1.

ASSESSING THE EFFECTS OF CHEMICALS ON HUMORAL IMMUNE FUNCTION

Loren D. Koller
School of Veterinary Medicine
University of Idaho
Moscow, ID 83843, USA

The immune system which is dispersed throughout the body of living organisms is composed of a myriad of cellular components which in unison interact in a balanced fashion. This complex system regulates body defense mechanisms by monitoring and responding to altered antigenic composition of the body. The regulatory events of the immune system are to: 1) distinguish, but not react with, normal antigens of the body; 2) identify foreign antigens such as microorganisms and neoplastic cells and successfully destroy and eliminate them from the body; and 3) maintain a delicate balance for optimum performance.

The immune system is regulated by multiple chemical signals operating at different levels. Antigens trigger local chemical signals which in turn trigger a network of responding cells operative throughout the body. The overall responsiveness of the system is controlled by modification of cellular components, their secretory products as well as signals from endocrine glands. Thymic hormones and corticosteroids in particular have immunoregulatory activities. Disruption of any one of these events not only impedes immunologic processes, but also results in diminished responses.

This report is concerned with one major component of the immune system, i.e., humoral immunity. The humoral immune system is relatively easy to measure. The B lymphocyte, the cell which confers humoral immunity, secretes antibody into the circulation which can be detected in the serum. Antibody titers can be measured by a multitude of immunoassays. This system is readily accessible to immunomodulation by chemicals. In addition, since humoral immune responses are frequently regulated by T lymphocytes, macrophages and/or their secretory products, altered humoral responses could be indicative of damage to these components as well as B-lymphocytes. In that sense, modulation of humoral immunity by chemicals could represent severe dysfunction indicative of damage to other segments of the immune system.

Two features of humoral immunity will be discussed. The first will be to briefly describe the ontogeny and regulatory characteristics of

NATO ASI Series, Vol. G2
Immunotoxicology. Edited by P. W. Mullen

B lymphocytes. The second will be to discuss methodology available to assess chemical induced modulation of humoral immunity.

CHARACTERISTICS OF HUMORAL IMMUNITY

B lymphocytes, as do other immune cells, arise from hematopoietic stem cells. Stem cells and precursor B cells replenish antigen sensitive B lymphocytes from bone marrow which is the primary site of continuous production and differentiation of immunoglobulin bearing small lymphocytes. These cells interact with each other and antigen to trigger differentiation which gives rise to plasma cells or memory B cells. The plasma cells produce and secrete antibody while the memory cells are responsible primarily for secondary responses.

B cells are identified by surface receptors. B lymphocytes bear membrane associated immunoglobulin (Buckley, 1976). B cells also have surface receptors for the activated third component (C3 receptor) of complement and for the Fc portions of IgG molecules. It is possible that B lymphocytes may also have receptors for macrophages and T cell factors.

Immunoglobulins (antibodies) are a group of glycoproteins closely related by structure and function. Five major classes of immunoglobulins (IgM, IgG, IgA, IgE, and IgD) have been identified on the basis of their physical, chemical, and antigenic properties (Eisen, 1974). The primary function of the antibody molecule is to selectively bind antigen. The amino acid sequence and spatial arrangement determine antigen specificity of the immunoglobulin. In general, however, it is the chemical structure of the antigen that actually determines the resulting specificity and affinity of the antibody molecule.

Another important feature in antigen-antibody reactions is avidity, i.e., the tendency of antibody to combine and form stable complexes with the antigen. Combination of antigen and antibody is specific and reversible. Therefore, there is continual dissociation of antigen and antibody in immune reactions.

There are essentially three stages of the humoral immune response: (1) triggering of B lymphocytes by antigen followed by, (2) proliferation, and, finally, (3) maturation and differentiation into plasma cells that synthesize and release antibody as well as memory B lymphocytes. The antibody response to many antigens requires cooperation between B and T cells and often macrophages. The association of these cells will be discussed later.

Introduction of antigen into a host results in either direct stimulation of B cells or the antigen may initially be "processed" by macrophages which transfer the antigenic determinants to B lymphocytes. The sensitized small lymphocytes progress through a series of transformations into large lymphocytes and finally lymphoblasts which differentiate into antibody secreting plasma cells or small memory lymphocytes.

The reaction commences when antigen molecules encounter small lymphocytes with surface antibody to that particular antigen. The antigen is bound to the antibody which provokes the small lymphocytes to divide and differentiate. During differentiation, the surface antigen-antibody complexes are lost and replaced by new antibody receptors. The memory cells possess surface immunoglobulin receptors similar to the original small lymphocytes while plasma cells synthesize and secrete circulating antibody.

Antigen can be destroyed in a variety of ways. Complement fixation may occur in some bacterial infections by provoking lysis (immune adherence) of the cell membrane. Other antigens stimulate production of antibodies which enhance phagocytosis (opsonic adherence). Another method is neutralization by antibody (or antitoxin) directed against a toxin. Once the toxin is controlled, the cells producing the toxin can be destroyed by phagocytosis.

The memory cell, on the other hand, is a resting antigen-sensitized B cell which responds to a second exposure to that antigen by rapid production of large amounts of antibody. These antibodies usually have a greater affinity and specificity for antigen than those produced after initial exposure.

The primary immune response represents the individual's first contact with a particular antigen. IgM appears early and is the principal antibody of the primary response but the response later shifts to IgG.

The secondary immune response (memory, anamnestic response) represents reexposure to the same antigen weeks, months, or even years after the primary antibody response has subsided. The antibody which is produced (primarily IgG) persists, has a prolonged steady state, and has a greater affinity for antigen than those produced during the primary response. IgG production is by far greater in the secondary response than primary response while IgM is similar for both responses.

Antibody responses to many antigens require cooperation between at least two types of lymphocytes for optimal expression. Differentiation of bone marrow derived B cells into antibody-secreting plasma cells is usually regulated by thymus-derived T cells. The function of the T cell and its soluble factors are not to produce antibody, but rather to aid in activation and proliferation of B cells (Janeway, 1975). A third cell type, the macrophage, also has an important role as an accessory cell by cooperating with T cells and aiding the response of B cells to antigens.

There are at least four types of T cells recognized to date. These include cytotoxic, helper, amplifier, and suppressor T cells. All but the cytotoxic lymphocyte function in regulating the humoral immune response. The helper T cell is required for activation of B cells to many antigens while the amplifier T cell regulates proliferation of activated B lymphocytes. This cooperation may occur either by cell to cell contact or by release of soluble factors by T cells (Yu and Gordon, 1973). The other T cell, suppressor T, is responsible for suppressing antibody synthesis by inhibiting B lymphocytes. In general, B cell activity is regulated by a balance of helper and suppressor T cells. Exposure to a weak or small antigen dose may induce helper T cells while a strong antigen or larger dose may induce suppressor T cells thereby controlling amount of antibody synthesized.

The IgG response is considerably more dependent on the helper T cell than is the IgM response (Anderson, Dresser and Wortis, 1974; Paraskeras and Lee, 1976). T cells are not necessary for induction of memory in B cells but T cells or soluble factors derived from activated T cells are important in expression of B memory upon rechallenge (Schrader, 1975; Lafrenz and Feldbush, 1981). Furthermore, a greater antibody response can occur if the number of antigen-activated T cells increases independently of B cells (Rowley, Fitch, Stuart, Kohler and Cosenza, 1973). These T cells circulate long after exposure to antigen and are thought to account in part for memory.

Macrophages are also modulators of humoral immunity. Macrophages, like B lymphocytes, have receptors for complement and the Fc portion of immunoglobulin. One function of macrophages is to localize and/or align antigen and bring it closer to an antibody-forming lymphocyte. Macrophages may also process antigen in lysosomes making it highly antigenic (Nakano and Muramatsu, 1976; Walker, 1976; Lipscomb, Ben-Sasson and Uhr, 1977). It is not exactly clear how the macrophage-antigen interaction results in enhanced antigen immunogenicity. It is known, however, that both antigen-induced lymphocyte proliferation and the differentiation of antibody-forming cells from lymphocyte precursors during the primary response _in vitro_ require the assistance of macrophages (Nielsen, Jensen, Braendstrup and Werdelin, 1974). Like the T-B cell interaction, this cooperation may occur by physical contact between the macrophage and B cell or by soluble factors released from the macrophage. Macrophages also activate T lymphocytes to produce nonspecific helper activity for antibody production (Erb and Feldman, 1975; Jackway, Thomas and Talmage, 1975).

ASSAYS TO MEASURE HUMORAL IMMUNITY

A myriad of assays have been used to assess humoral immunity. Some of them include measurement of antibody titers (immunodiffusion, complement fixation, serum neutralization, hemagglutination, passive hemagglutination, radioimmunoassay, enzyme-linked immunosorbent assay, etc.), antibody synthesis (Jerne and Cunningham plaque assay, Mishell-Dutton techniques), polyclonal activation (*Escherichia coli* lipopolysaccharide), B lymphocyte receptors (Fc and complement), and memory responses. Some of these procedures are amenable to assessment of both *in vivo* and *in vitro* exposures to chemicals.

Humoral immunity may be determined after initial exposure to the antigen (primary response) or after re-challenge with antigen (secondary or memory response). Staining of surface immunoglobulin will identify B lymphocytes and enumerate percent B cells. Many antigens, both T-dependent and T-independent, have been utilized in these investigations. Some of these antigens are tetanus toxoid, sheep red blood cells, bovine serum albumin, ovalbumin, bovine gammaglobulin, *Salmonella typhi*, pseudorabies virus, influenza virus, keyhole limpet hemocyanin and lipopolysaccharide.

Polyclonal activators (mitogens) can induce blast transformation of normal lymphocytes. *Escherichia coli* lipopolysaccharide (LPS) stimulates B lymphocytes while pokeweed mitogen (PWM) activates both T and B lymphocytes. Interference of B blastogenesis may indicate humoral involvement. However, polyclonal activators do not necessarily reflect immune function since they only provoke cell division and DNA synthesis. Since the degree of mitogen stimulation is regulated by macrophages, the ratio of macrophages to lymphocytes in culture must be standardized. The usefulness of mitogens was recently questioned since altered responses usually occur only in the presence of extremely severe abnormalities (Blakley and Archer, 1982).

The humoral immune system can best be evaluated by development of highly sensitive, reproducible, and quantitative assays which measure antibody. Several methods are available to measure antibody titers in serum. However, two of the most recently developed assays, radioimmunoassay (RIA) and enzyme-linked immunosorbent assay (ELISA), appear to have considerable application to assess immunotoxicity of chemicals. The characteristics of these two techniques qualify as representative assays for humoral immunity. The versatility of the ELISA method, for instance, allows for measurement of antigens, haptens, or antibodies. Other advantages of this technique are its sensitivity for detection of specific antibodies, reproducibility, and potential for large scale screening due to automation of practically all analytical steps.

Furthermore, because only a very small sample of blood is required for testing, the same animal can be sampled periodically during a long term experiment thus requiring fewer animals and reducing costs.

Data obtained from the ELISA can be reported by several methods such as: (1) an absorbance value (405 nm) at one specific dilution of serum; (2) the absorbance for series of dilutions of serum presented in tabular or graphic form; (3) an endpoint serum dilution at which absorbance drops below the blank; or (4) as actual mg of antibody per ml of serum by extrapolation to a normal curve prepared by analyzing serial dilutions of a similar antibody of known concentrations (Koller, Exon, Moore and Watanabe, submitted for publication). The format of listing absorbance values for a series of serum dilutions is most informative and less subjective to misinterpretation which may result from comparison of data at only one serum dilution or an endpoint dilution. The former format will reveal major differences in slope of the titration curves in addition to the endpoint. The data are further enhanced if reported as actual mg antibody per ml of serum.

The endpoint of the ELISA is indicative of the amount of specific antibodies which are elicited and are present in the serum. Alteration of antibody levels in the serum could result from impairment of several intermediary pathways (e.g., helper or suppressor T cell function, processing and presentation of antigen by macrophages, protein synthesis, etc.) which could be determined by more specific assays, if desired.

The Jerne plaque technique (Jerne and Nordin, 1963) and modifications by Cunningham and Szenberg (1968) can be utilized to assess antibody synthesis. These assays determine the actual number of cells which produce antibody. The value of these procedures is to distinguish if modulation of the immune response occurs intracellularly or from catabolism of the antibody molecule once it has been synthesized. The technique also delineates between the primary (IgM) and secondary (IgG) immune response.

A hemolytic antibody isotope release (HAIR) assay was recently developed which is an alternative to the conventional plaque assays (Steppen and Kerkvliet, 1981). This technique measures the amount of antibody produced by the splenic plaque-forming cells and a significant correlation occurred between the results obtained from the HAIR assay and standard plaque-forming techniques.

The EA and EAC rosette assays measure activity of Fc and complement receptors, respectively, on the surface of B lymphocytes. Alteration of receptor activity on B cells could result in impaired immune function of that cell. These techniques detect specific responses and discern mechanistic features of lymphocyte function.

Re-exposure to certain antigens may occur weeks or even months after initial exposure. This is particularly important in revaccination programs since production of antibody for the secondary immune response depends on activity of a memory cell which develops after initial antigen exposure. Diminished memory activity would contribute to a reduced secondary antibody response while the primary response may be affected more by direct involvement of the B lymphocytes or perhaps impediment of helper T cells or augmentation of suppressor T cells which regulate the function of B lymphocytes.

A model in vitro system for growth of lymphocytes in culture was developed by Mishell and Dutton (1967). This system provides adequate conditions for in vitro immunization which closely parallels in vivo responses. The procedure has application to manipulate cell populations in vitro to assess chemical insult to specific cell types and subsets. Further, immune cells can be exposed to the chemical either in vivo or in vitro. This technique adds another dimension to the immunotoxicologists' repertoire to delineate chemical perturbations of the humoral immune system.

The recent development of monoclonal antibodies should have a marked impact on immunotoxicology (Kohler and Milstein, 1975). Clones secreting large amounts of a single antibody molecule can be formed by the fusion of normal antibody-producing cells with (myeloma) tumor cells. Hybridoma is the term used for this combination. Monoclonal antibodies have been used in: methods for determining the fine structure of proteins, radioimmunoassay of hormones and drugs, histocompatibility testing, cancer detection, purification of molecules, immunotherapy, and have proven invaluable in distinguishing previously unidentified molecules, such as new surface antigens on subpopulations of lymphocytes.

In summary, the pathway of the humoral immune system from antigen stimulation to antibody synthesis is extremely complex. The B lymphocyte is the progenitor of antibody-forming plasma cells but optimum responses are not usually achieved without participation by T lymphocytes and macrophages. Furthermore, it is a balance between helper T and suppressor T as well as amplifier T and macrophages that regulate B cell activity and consequently the humoral immune response. The major identifiable property of humoral immunity is the production and secretion of antibody by lymphocytes.

Reliable, quantitative assays are currently available to delineate humoral immunity in animals which have been exposed to chemicals. These procedures are acceptable and accessible for use by industry and academia. However, researchers must be provoked to constantly improve methodology and remain progressive and creative to achieve and maintain "State of the Art" (monoclonal antibody, etc.) technology in all immunotoxicological investigations.

REFERENCES

ANDERSON, H.R., DRESSER, D.W. and WORTIS, H.H. (1974) The relationship between the immunoglobulin class of B-cell precursors and the degree of synergism obtained from the presence of T cells. Clin. Exp. Immunol., 16, 393.

BLAKLEY, B.R. and ARCHER, D.L. (1982) Mitogen stimulation of lymphocytes exposed to lead. Toxicol. Appl. Pharmacol., 62, 183.

BUCKLEY, R.H. (1976) The functions and measurement of human B and T lymphocytes. J. Invest. Dermatol., 67, 381.

CUNNINGHAM, A.J. and SZENBERG, A. (1968) Further improvements in the plaque technique for detecting single antibody-forming cells. Immunol., 14, 599.

EISEN, H.N. (1974) Immunology, Harper and Row Publishers, Hagerstown, MD, 460 and 512.

ERB, P. and FELDMAN, M. (1975) The role of macrophages in the generation of T helper cells. Eur. J. Immunol., 5, 759.

JACKWAY, J.P., THOMAS, D.W. and TALMAGE, D.W. (1975) Activation of T lymphocyte helper function by brief exposure to antigen-pulsed macrophages. Proc. Soc. Exp. Biol. Med., 150, 791.

JANEWAY, C.A. (1975) Cellular cooperation during in vivo anti-hapten antibody responses. I. The effect of cell number on the response. J. Immunol., 114, 1394.

JERNE, N.K. and NORDIN, A.A. (1963) Plaque formation in agar by single antibody-producing cells. Science, 140, 405.

KOHLER, G. and MILSTEIN, G. (1975) Continuous cultures of fused cells secreting antibody of predefined specificity. Nature, 256, 495.

KOLLER, L.D., EXON, J.H., MOORE, S.A. and WATANABE, P.G. (submitted for publication) Evaluation of ELISA for detecting in vivo chemical immunomodulation.

LAFRENZ, D.E. and FELDBUSH, T.L. (1981) Role of T cells in the development of memory B cells. Quantitative and qualitative analysis. Immunol., 44, 177.

LIPSCOMB, M.F., BEN-SASSON, S.Z. and UHR, J.W. (1977) Specific binding of T lymphocytes to macrophages. I. Kinetics of binding. J. Immunol., 118, 1748.

MISHELL, R.I. AND DUTTON, R.W. (1967) Immunization of dissociated spleen cell cultures from normal mice. J. Exp. Med. 126, 423.

NAKANO, K. and MURAMATSU, S. (1976) Studies on the role of macrophages in the antibody response of mice: Stimulation of T cell-dependent antibody responses by tolerogenic soluble antigen trapped by macrophages. J. Reticuloendothel. Soc., 19, 347.

NIELSEN, M.H., JENSEN, H., BRAENDSTRUP, O. and WERDELIN, Q. (1974) Macrophage-lymphocyte clusters in the immune response to soluble protein antigen _in vitro_. _J. Exp. Med._, _140_, 1260.

PARASKERAS, F. and LEE, S.T. (1976) The helper cell function of primed T cells. _Eur. J. Immunol._, _6_, 856.

ROWLEY, D.A. FITCH, F.W., STUART, F.P., KOHLER, H. and COSENZA, H. (1973) Specific suppression of immune responses. _Science_, _181_, 1133.

SCHRADER, J.W. (1975) The role of T cells in IgG production; thymus-dependent antigens induce B cell memory in the absence of T cells. _J. Immunol._, _114_, 1665.

STEPPAN, L.B. and KERKVLIET, N.I. (1981) The haemolytic antibody isotope release (HAIR) assay: An efficient alternative technique to conventional plaque assays. _Clin. Exp. Immunol._, _44_, 440.

WALKER, W.S. (1976) Functional heterogenicity of macrophages in the induction and expression of acquired immunity. _J. Reticuloendothel. Soc._, _20_, 57.

YU, H. and GORDON, J. (1973) Helper function in antibody synthesis mediated by soluble factors. _Nature (London) New Biol._, _244_, 20.

IMMUNE CELLS AND THEIR MODULATION BY EXOGENOUS SUBSTANCES

F. Spreafico, A. Vecchi, M. Sironi,
W. Luini, A. Canegrati, A. Merendino,
M. Allegrucci, M. Romano, I.E.F. Colotta

Istituto di Ricerche Farmacologiche "Mario Negri",
Via Eritrea 62, 20157 Milano, Italy

To the perceptive reader, a general conclusion clearly emerging from various chapters of this volume is that one has to regard the hybrid subspecialty of immunotoxicology as still in its halcyon days, (i.e. in a period of its evolution in which the number of problems already resolved is outweighed by those still open). In attempting to redress this balance, it seems appropriate to first examine what lessons concerning the immunological effects of xenobiotics in general can be learned from experience accumulated over the past two decades using agents employed primarily in therapeutic immunomodulation. Against this background, our experience in the evaluation of a series of immunotoxic substances shall be briefly reviewed with a view to extracting from this experience a number of aspects which appear to have greater general significance and application.

THERAPEUTIC IMMUNOMODULATORS AS MODEL COMPOUNDS IN IMMUNOTOXICOLOGY

As implied in the title of this section, since the focus will be centered on selected points possessing in our view more direct relevance to immunotoxicology, no attempt will here be made to discuss exhaustively the current state of the art of therapeutic non-specific immunomodulatory drugs *per se*. Indeed, the *heterogeneity* of these agents in terms of their effect on the various cellular components of the immune system is the single characteristic of particular relevance to the development of rationally based approaches to immunotoxicological assessment. (Even within the subcategory of immunosuppressive agents, heterogeneity of drug action is common.) Essentially, the general point we wish to emphasize is that not only immunocytes of different lineages vary in their susceptibility to the effect of cytotoxic agents employed in immunodepressive treatment, but that significant differences.

NATO ASI Series, Vol. G2
Immunotoxicology. Edited by P. W. Mullen

in this susceptibility can also be observed among subsets of a given population of immune cells. Furthermore, this heterogeneity in the qualitative-quantitative interaction with immunocytes by immunodepressants can be recognized also among agents possessing similar general modes of biochemical interference at the cell level and, indeed, among agents having close similarities in their chemical structure. An illustrative example of this complexity is presented in Table 1, which schematically summarizes studies using compounds representative of the main classes of cytotoxic drugs, on a number of mouse immunocytes. Taking into account the fact that macrophages and NK cells are currently

Table 1 Effect of chemical immunodepressants on the expression in murine spleen of macrophage and NK cell-mediated cytotoxicity and of T-dependent specific suppressive activity for humoral (abs) and cell-mediated (dth) reactivity to a T-dependent stimulus.

Compound	Macrophages	NK	Ts-abs		Ts-dth	
			progenit.	induced	progenit.	induced
Cyclophosphamide	=	=	↓↓↓	↓	↓	↓↓↓
Azathioprine	↓↓↓	↓↓↓	=	↓	=	=
Doxorubicin	=	=	↓↓↓	↓↓↓	↓↓↓	↓↓↓
Daunorubicin	↓↓↓	↓↓↓	=	=	↓↓	↓↓

= indicates no effect

given the main role in sustaining host natural resistance towards infections and neoplastic development, a first point illustrated by these results is that chemicals, even if employed in doses giving comparable depression of standard immune reactivities, can differ with respect to the effects exerted on specific cell types. Such findings may have relevance in connection with the choice of host-resistance assays for the immunotoxicological screening of unknown compounds. The possibility that chemicals closely related structurally, possessing identical acute and chronic general toxicity and believed to exert their cytotoxicity through common molecular mechanisms, can nevertheless drastically differ in important aspects of their immunological activity, is illustrated by the dissimilar effects of doxorubicin and daunorubicin on macrophages and NK cells. It should be noted that the contrasting effects on macrophages seen after *in vivo* treatment with these two anthracyclines, whose main mode of action is generally attributed to DNA intercalation, are not limited only to the expression of cytotoxic capacity but extends also to all other functional capacities of these cells, and can be observed in vitro on mature non-replicating elements of this series. This finding is illustrative of the fact that even in the case of antireplicative drugs as those mainly considered in this section, one should not look at the basis of their immunological activity solely in terms of the consequences of their inhibition of cell multiplication within the lymphoid system. As discussed more at length elsewhere (Spreafico and Anaclerio, 1977; Spreafico and Mantovani, 1981; Spreafico, Tagliabue and Vecchi, 1983; Spreafico, Alberti, Allegrucci, Canegrati, Colotta, Luini, Pasqueletto, Romano, Sironi and Vecchi, 1983a), there are in fact indications that the immunological mode of action of various immunodepressants also involves non-lethal modifications of cell functional capacity and/or maturational ability, as for instance represented by interference with production or responsiveness to interleukins. To further emphasize the possibility that proliferation-independent mechanisms can also be affected by antiproliferative compounds although through molecular mechanisms in most cases still hypothetical, Table 2 schematically lists the effects exerted by various immunodepressants on different aspects of macrophage physiology of direct relevance in immunity. The possibility

Table 2 Possible levels of interference of xenobiotics with cells of the monocyte-macrophage series.

- Interference with production-maturation (e.g. (+)Azathioprine, Corticosteroids)
- Killing of mature cells (e.g. (+)Daunorubicin;(-)Doxorubicin)
- Interference with functional capacity
  - antigen processing-phagocytosis (e.g. (+)Steroids, Vinca alkaloids)
  - expression of direct cytotoxicity (e.g.(+) Daunorubicin, 5FU, Steroids;(-)Vinca alkaloids, Cyclophosphamide, Doxorubicin)
  - expression of antibody-dependent cytotoxicity (e.g. (+)Cyclophosphamide; (-)Doxorubicin)
  - sensitivity to cytokines (e.g.(+) Steroids, Methotrexate, Azathioprine)
  - migration capacity (e.g.(+) Azathioprine, Vinca alkaloids)

(+) indicates an effective compound
(-) indicates an ineffective compound

on the other hand, that within a given population of immunocytes, there exists subsets of cells within a specific organ which differ in their susceptibility to foreign compounds is exemplified by the data of Table 1, in which the effects of *in vivo* treatment with various agents on the expression of T-dependent specific suppressive activity are summarized. Using a murine model condition in which specific suppressor cells (Ts) were induced by overstimulation with sheep erythrocytes, it was in fact observed that the expression of specific suppression for cellular responses to this antigen was differently affected by various drugs given before or after the Ts-inducing stimulus. In addition, the susceptibility to drugs of the expression of suppression for cellular responses differed from that of suppression for humoral responses to the same antigen. It should be noted in this connection that differences in the sensitivity of subsets within the same general population of immunocytes have been observed also with other drugs (Spreafico, Tagliabue and Vecchi, 1983). For instance, cyclophosphamide (Cy) has been shown to be relatively ineffective on T cells mediating allogeneic cytotoxicity while being very depressive of T-dependent, H-2 restricted cytotoxicity (Hurme, 1979). Similarly, cyclosporin A administration to rodents decreased spleen lymphocyte responsiveness to PHA while totally sparing that to ConA (Alberti, Boraschi, Luini and Tagliabue, 1981). On a more general level, the examples of heterogenous sensitivity to chemicals observable not only among cells of different lineages but also within cells of a given series, imply that foreign compounds can markedly vary in their effects on the immune complex, with the possibility that even molecules closely similar to one another may exibit quite distinct immunotoxicological profiles not only in quantitative but also qualitative terms.

Evaluation of xenobiotics' effects on immune cells is generally performed on certain cells of "central" compartments, such as blood or spleen. Since evidence has been obtained showing that in various species including man at least certain types of immunocytes vary substantially in their physiological capacity depending on their anatomical site of residence (Walker, 1976; Mantovani, Biondi, Introna, Bottazzi, Polentarutti and Bordignon, 1982), the question can be raised as to whether immunocytes present in different organs vary in their modulability by exogenous compounds. This question has obvious relevance considering that real-life exposure to xenobiotics can be expected to involve, at least initially, peripheral organs such as the lung or intestine, which are rich in certain types of immune cells and/or are the site of specialized immune subsystems (e.g. the gut). The possibility that indeed the functional capacity of immunocytes present in different lymphoid and non-lymphoid organs may be differently affected by given xenobiotics is illustrated in Table 3 which summarizes a series of recent results detailed elsewhere (Spreafico <u>et al</u>, 1983a). Thus for instance, the parenteral administration to mice of 5-fluorouracil (5-FU) was associated with significant depressions of macrophage capacity to express non-specific cytotoxicity in the lung and peritoneal cavity but not in the spleen despite the use of doses capable of clearly depressing antibody-producing splenocytes. Similarly, parenteral injection of

Table 3 Effect of immunodepressants on the functional activity of immunocytes in different organs.

Drug	Route	macrophages			NK			Con A		PHA	
		spleen	perit.	lung	spleen	lung	gut	blood	spleen	blood	spleen
Cy	iv-ip	=	↓	=	↓	↓	↓	↓	↓	↓	↓
Aza	sc-ip	↓	↓	=	↓	=	=	↓	=	↓	=
5Fu	ip-os	=	↓	↓	↓	↓	↑	=	=	↓	=
DxR	iv	=	=	=	=	=	=	=	=	=	=
OHcort	sc-ip	↓		↓	↓	↓	=	↓	↓		

= indicates no effect

↓ indicates a decrease

↑ indicates an increase

azathioprine (Aza) reduced the functional capacity of macrophages taken from spleen and peritoneum but not from the lung, thus exhibiting an organ-related preferentiality in inducing macrophage damage not observed conversely with compounds such as hydrocortisone which decreased macrophage function at all sites considered. Table 3 shows that an organ-associated preferentiality in the modulation exerted on a given type of immune cell was not restricted only to macrophages. Single parenteral doses of Aza induced clear reductions in NK activity in the spleen but not in lung and gut, whereas hydrocortisone (OH-cort.) was depressive of this capacity in spleen and lung but not in the intestine. Injection of 5FU was associated with evident decreases in spleen and lung NK activity concomitantly with very marked increases in the capacity of intestinal intraepithelial lymphoid cells to express the same activity, a finding in turn due to inhibition at this site of the cells down-regulating NK activity. Conversely, Cy was depressed and doxorubicin (DXR) spared NK activity at each of the three sites investigated. Lastly,

Table 3 shows that whereas some chemicals exerted parallel effects on the T-mitogen responsiveness of cells taken from blood and spleen, discordant results were seen with other compounds, such as Aza and 5FU.

The basis for the selectivity exhibited by drugs vis-a-vis the different populations and subsets of immunocytes is by and large still hypothetical. Similarly unresolved are the mechanisms responsible for the different susceptibilities to a given drug of cells of the same type present in different organs. A correlation between drug concentrations and their effect in different organs has been observed for some agents (e.g. in the case of hydrocortisone activity on NK activity in spleen, lung and intestine). However, such correlations were not seen with other agents and the importance of differences in compound bioavailability at various sites relative to other possible mechanisms (e.g. inter-organ differences in turnover rates of cells; intrinsic differences in susceptibility to damage or repair) is still very much an open problem, in view of the distinct possibility that different mechanisms may operate and interact for different compounds. Regardless of the operative mechanisms accounting for the differential susceptibility of immunocytes present in different sites to modulation by xenobiotics, these findings raise the possibility that effects measured at "central" organs may not be representative of what occurs at other more peripheral locations, such as lung and gut which represent first line barriers against the external milieu, and where the initial encounter between host and xenobiotic actually takes place. The importance of using realistic routes of exposure in the evaluation of the potential immunotoxicity of xenobiotics is, of course, a key consideration.

EXPERIENCE WITH SELECTED IMMUNOACTIVE XENOBIOTICS

As already mentioned, the aim of this section is to extract from our experience concerning the immune effects of various compounds, a number of characteristics of possible more general significance. We refer therefore to other publications for more detailed descriptions and discussions of the data briefly summarized herein (Spreafico, Vecchi, Mantovani, Tagliabue, Sironi, Luini and Garattini, 1981b; Spreafico and Vecchi, 1983).

As an example of the fact that xenobiotics may reveal preferential, if not true selective effects, on different populations and subpopulations of immune cells, we shall first consider the steroid contraceptive agents (Vecchi, Tagliabue, Mantovani, 1976; Spreafico, Vecchi, Anaclerio, Moras, Tagliabue, Barale, Mantovani, Sironi and Polentarutti, 1977) bearing in mind that much of what we have learned about therapeutic immunodepressants also applies to immunotoxic compounds. The immunological activity of these synthetic steroids, as summarized in Table 4, clearly reveals that the immunodepression associated with their administration to rodents is exerted selectively via T-cell dependent reactivities, whereas the functional capacity of B cells is unaffected. This is typically revealed by the finding that the response to T-independent antigens and

Table 4 Steroid contraceptives and immune reactivity in rodents.

T dependent reactivities	↓ abs titers to T-dependent ags; ↓ EAE; ↓autoabs titres; ↓ ConA; ↓$Thyl^+$ cell numbers
B dependent reactivities	= abs titres to T-independent ags; = LPS = B cell numbers

↓ indicates a decrease
= indicates no change
(abs = antibody; ags = antigen)

B mitogens is normal after treatments capable of significantly reducing reactivity to T mitogens, T-dependent antigens, or in models of T-dependent diseases such as experimental allergic encephalomyelitis (EAE). It may also be worth noting that steroid contraceptives-induced immunodepression appears to be associated with reduced proportions of T but not B cells in lymphoid organs, although total cellularity in these tissues is not significantly modified. Since the doses of contraceptives employed in these investigations were the minimal ones giving 100% antifertility effects in rodents (i.e. realistic, rather than suprapharmacological treatments were used), it appears that the animal data have relevance to the human situation. In fact, it has been reported that in women on "The Pill", improvements in autoimmune conditions and reduced autoantibody levels may occur along with decreased mitogen responsiveness and responses to standard vaccines (Royal College of Practitioners, 1974).

Since cells of the T lineage are believed to be more important in the resistance to viral challenges, the higher incidence of viral infections described in Third World populations receiving oral contraceptives (Royal College of Practitioners, 1974), appears to lend support to the animal data. The absence of augmented rates of infections in Western World users of the Pill could be explained considering that in animals the immunodepression observed is relatively moderate and recovers quickly upon discontinuation of treatment. Relatively minor pre-existing derangements (subclinical *per se*), could combine with other immunomodifying factors (e.g. endemic viral presence, low protein-calorie nutrition), thus resulting in clear pathological effects. Relevant to this point and the possibility discussed in the preceding section that substances of the same pharmacological class may vary in their immunopharmacological or -toxicological profile, is the fact that clear quantitative differences in immunodepressive capacities were seen among the contraceptive estroprogestinic combinations studied even when employed at equally effective anti-fertility doses.

A brief discussion of the immunological activity of the plant proteins MCI and PAP-S serves to illustrate two concepts of some general relevance in immunotoxicology, namely that natural substances can also affect immunity, and that xenobiotics' activity on the cells of the immune system can be very complex as manifested by the simultaneous presence of opposite effects on different cell types. MCI and PAP-S, which are 30,000 dalton proteins extracted from the seeds of *Momordica charantia* and *Phytolaica americana*, respectively, are representative of a group of similar proteins widely distributed in the plant kingdom, which bear a number of close structural and biochemical resemblances to the A-chain of ricin. The A-chain is the part of the ricin molecule which irreversibly binds and inactivates ribosomes, whereas the B-chain, absent in MIC and PAP-S, binds to the cell membrane. As summarized in Table 5, MCI and PAP-S are powerful immunodepressants when administered parenterally to rodents, this effect involving selectively cells of the T lineage, B cells being significantly more resistant *in vitro* and *in vivo* to both proteins. At the same time, however, these substances, at otherwise strongly immunodepressive doses, induce *in vitro* and *in vivo* a very powerful augmentation in the expression of macrophage-dependent cytotoxicity (Spreafico, Malfiore, Moras, Marmonti, Filippeschi, Barbieri, Perocco and Stirpe, 1983b). Although the mechanistic basis for this set of apparently contrasting effects induced by MCI and PAP-S is still unclear, it seems important to emphasize that a large body of evidence now exists in support of the fact that both immunodepressants and stimulators can induce a variety of paradoxical effects ranging from the simultaneous presence at the same dose of enhancement of certain immune functions and depression in others, to changes in the direction of the modification induced, depending on the dose employed (Spreafico, 1980; Spreafico, Vecchi, Conti and Sironi, 1981a). Although in the context of immunotoxicity much more attention has traditionally been paid to the "depressive" consequences of exposure to xenobiotics, it should be strongly emphasized that derangement in any direction away from physiological equilibrium should be regarded as potentially harmful.

Table 5 Effects on immune reactivity of the plant proteins MCI and PAP-S

T cells :	↓-SRBC PFC numbers; ↓-SRBC DTH; ↓ allograft rejection ↓ response to Con A-PHA (*in vitro* and *in vivo*)
B cells :	= PFC numbers to T-independent ags; = response to LPS mitogen (*in vitro* and *in vivo*)
NK cells :	↓ expression of cytotoxicity
Macrophages :	↑ expression of cytotoxicity (*in vitro* and *in vivo*)

↓ indicates decrease

↑ indicates increase

= indicates no change

In other words, to be considered immunotoxic, a substance needs not to induce solely immunodepressive effects considering in addition that, as exemplified above, the cells sustaining the various specific and non-specific regulatory networks existing within the immune system are not intrinsically resistant to modulation or killing by exogenous compounds. Thus, immunodepression can be the consequence of an "activation" of suppressor elements, whereas their inactivation can result in a condition of partial, or complete, enhancement of immune function.

In view of the fact that the immunological activity of polyhalogenated dibenzodioxins, such as TCDD, has already been described in detail by this and other groups (Vos and Moore, 1974; Luster, Faith and Clark, 1979; Mantovani, Vecchi, Luini, Sironi, Candiani, Spreafico and Garattini, 1980; Vecchi, Mantovani, Sironi, Luini, Spreafico and Garattini, 1980; Vos, Faith and Luster, 1980; Vecchi, Sironi, Canegrati and Garattini, 1983), we shall here emphasize only a few aspects of the experimental immunotoxicology of 2,3,7,8-tetrachlorodibenzoparadioxin (TCDD). The first point of practical relevance to immunotoxicological screening generally is the fact that the degree of humoral depression induced by TCDD in mice is markedly strain-dependent, a finding which is attributable to the existance of inter-strain variations in the number and/or affinity of the specific binding sites for this chemical present in lymphoid and non-lymphoid cells. For instance, a dose of 1.2μg/kg TCDD causing more than 70% reduction in the number of primary anti-sheep erythrocyte antibody-producing splenocytes in C57Bl/6 mice, is totally ineffective in animals of the DBA/2 strain. The existence of variations amongst strains as well as between species, with respect to susceptibility to exogenously-induced immunomodulation with a number of compounds, implies that more than one animal species should be employed in immunotoxicological testing if one intends to provide meaningful extrapolations to man. A second point of some general methodological interest emerging from the TCDD investigations, is that on a unit cell number basis, no reduction in macrophage and NK cell functional capacity was seen in young adult mice given immunodepressive TCDD doses. However, since the chemical induced lymphoid cell depletion, the total organ capacity to mediate macrophage and NK cell-dependent activities was in effect reduced. This point deserves specific mention in view of the frequent tendency to investigate xenobiotics' effects on single immunocyte types without considering the total context in which the cells are physiologically present. Although TCDD administration to adult rodents is not associated with significant decreases in macrophage and NK cell functional ability, a clear reduction in both is conversely seen when exposure to the compound occurs during pregnancy or in the early post-partum period, an impairment compounding that attributable to lymphoid cell depletion. As pre- or perinatal exposure to TCDD results in a greater depression also of other types of immune reactivity, this chemical serves as a good example of the fact that the developing immune system is in general, more sensitive to pertubation by exogenous substances than is the mature one. An enhanced susceptibility can also be expected to exist during aging of the immune system. This point should be given special attention in both the investigational and safety evaluation of several different categories of immunotoxins which might involve not only healthy adults but also individuals at both age extremes, in whom additional subthreshold or overt causes for immune derangement may co-exist. Unfortunately, such considerations and a realization that in real life xenobiotic exposure involves not a single chemical but mixtures with the consequent possibility of complex interactions, are not normally considered in immunotoxicological (indeed, in general toxicological) testing.

As discussed elsewhere (Spreafico and Vecchi, 1983), various points should be considered when attempting to define an immunotoxic substance, such as the use in testing of realistic conditions of exposure including dose and its route of administration — key considerations which are obviously crucial to the problem of animal-man extrapolation. In this connection, data obtained (Spreafico et al, 1981b) in the course of investigating the possible immunological effects of the synthetic sweetener saccharin may be illustrative (Table 6). The administration for 30 days to rats and mice of saccharin in the diet at concentrations above 1% was associated with evident reductions in primary humoral antibody formation, while T-dependent and macrophage or NK cell mediated reactivities as well as lymphoid organ cellularity were unaffected. As this chemical is not metabolized *in vivo*, *in vitro* tests can also be informative. Thus, *in vitro*, while macrophages and NK cell functions were unaltered, the response of lymphocytes to T and B mitogens was consistantly reduced at saccharin concentrations of 1-2mg/ml whereas no effects were seen at lower concentrations. However, comparing the bioavailability parameters of saccharin in rats and man it was shown that the peak levels reached in the serum of rats given an immunodepressive saccharin diet are approximately two orders of magnitude higher than those attainable in humans given the normal average daily intake of this chemical, a finding which should be considered in light of the relatively steep dose-response curve for saccharin-associated immune

Table 6 Saccharin and immune parameters.

in vitro (0.5mg/ml)	= macrophage function; = NK cell function; = mitogen response in both murine and human lymphocytes; = mitogen response in human
in vivo (1-5% diet in rodents)	= macrophage function; = NK cell function; - SRBC PFC numbers; - SRBC DTH

= indicates no effect
- indicates a decrease

effects in animals. It is well established that bioavailability data based on the concentrations in body fluids and/or target organs of the chemical or its biologically active biotransformation products represent a more correct approach for these interspecies comparisons than simple comparisons of doses administered. Of relevance not only to the specific extrapolation of saccharin animal data to humans but also to immunotoxicity in general, is the finding that the mitogen responsiveness of human lymphocytes *in vitro* was totally resistant to saccharin concentrations capable of profoundly inhibiting the same response in rodent cells. Such findings serve as a further reminder that interspecies comparisons should take into account not only the possibility of the existence of significant differences in metabolism and tissue distribution of chemicals, but additionally that intrinsic differences in sensitivity to damage may exist between animal and human immunocytes. Notwithstanding the many limitations of in vitro testing, the possibility of analysing in tissue culture a number of immune functions with easily obtained human cells provides immunotoxicology with a distinct advantage over other types of toxicological testing.

CONCLUSION

It is now abundantly clear that there exists a large number of substances which, by virtue of their selectivity in exerting damage to the immune system compared to other organ systems, can rightly be regarded as immunotoxic. In addition, immunotoxicity is a property of certain xenobiotics which shows considerable variations with respect to its cause, nature and underlying biological phenomena. As expected, considering the complexity of the immune system and thus the vast number of possible levels and mechanisms whereby damage can be exerted, immunotoxic compounds represent a composite category of substances in terms of the types of immune effects displayed. This heterogeneity has obvious conceptual and practical implications at different levels and is an important factor to be taken into account in the future formulation of the basic principles and tenets of immunotoxicology. Hybrid sub-specialities such as immunotoxicology frequently experience difficulties in their launching because of the problems in properly integrating the different disciplines involved. However, the number of compounds having immunotoxic potential and their often widespread distribution in the human environment, together with the realization of the crucial role of a well balanced immune system in health maintenance, will undoubtedly act as an impetus for us to strive for the full manifestations of the potential "hybrid vigor" inherent in this important interdisciplinary science.

ACKNOWLEDGEMENT

This work was supported in part by grant no. 81.01747.95 "Progetto Finalizzato Chimica Fine Secondaria", CNR, Rome.

REFERENCES

ALBERTI, S., BORASCHI, D., LUINI, W. and TAGLIABUE, A. (1981) Effects of in vivo treatments with cyclosporin A on mouse cell-mediated immune responses. Int. J. Immunopharmac. 3, 357.

HURME, M. (1979) Differential cyclophosphamide sensitivity of precursor cells in allogeneic and H-2 restricted cytotoxic responses. J. Exp. Med. 149, 290.

LUSTER, M.I., FAITH, R.E. and CLARK, G. (1979) Laboratory studies on the immune effects of halogenated aromatics. Ann. N.Y. Acad. Sci. 320, 473.

MANTOVANI, A., BIONDI, A., INTRONA, M., BOTTAZZI, B., POLENTARUTTI, N. and BORDIGNON, C. (1982) Human macrophage population with different tumoricidal and immunoregulatory activity. Functional status of tumor-associated inflammatory cells. p. 257. In: Current Concepts in Human Immunology and Cancer Immunomodulation. (eds. Serrou, B., Rosenfeld, c., daniels, J.C. and Saunders, J.P.) Elsevier, Amsterdam.

MANTOVANI, A., VECCHI, A., LUINI, W., SIRONI, M., CANDIANI, G.P., SPREAFICO, F. and GARATTINI, S. (1980) Effect of 2,3,7,8-tetrachloro-dibenzo-p-dioxin on macrophage and natural killer cell-mediated cyto-toxicity in mice. Biomedicine 32, 200.

ROYAL COLLEGE OF PRACTITIONERS (1974) A Report of the Oral Contraceptive Study. Pitman Medical Publications, London.

SPREAFICO, F. (1980) Current problems with immunopotentiating agents. p. 189. In: The Immune System: Functions and Therapy of Dysfunction. (eds. Doria, G. and Eshkol, A.) Academic Press, London.

SPREAFICO, F., ALBERTI, S., ALLEGRUCCI, M., CANEGRATI, A., COLOTTA, F., LUINI, W., PASQUALETTO, E., ROMANO, M., SIRONI, M. and VECCHI, A. (1983a) On the mode of action of immunodepressant agents. In: Advances in Immunopharmacology 2. (eds. Hadden, J.W., Chedid, L., Dukor, P., Spreafico, F. and Willoughby, D.) Pergamon Press, Oxford.

SPREAFICO, F. and ANACLERIO, A. (1977) Immunosuppressive agents. p. 245. In: Immunopharmacology. (eds. Hadden, J.W., Coffey, R.G. and Spreafico, F.) Plenum Press, New York.

SPREAFICO, F., MALFIORE, C., MORAS, M.L., MARMONTI, L., FILIPPESCHI, S., BARBIERI, L., PEROCCO, P. and STIRPE, F. (1983b) The immunomodulatory activity of the plant proteins Momordica Charantia inhibitor and pokeweed antiviral protein. Int. J. Immunopharmac. 5, 335.

SPREAFICO, F. and MANTOVANI, A. (1981) Immunomodulation by cancer chemotherapeutic agents and antineoplastic activity, p. 177. In: Pathobiology Annual 1981. (ed. Ioachim, H.L.) Raven Press, New York.

SPREAFICO, F., TAGLIABUE, A. and VECCHI, A. (1983c) Chemical immuno-depressant . In: Immunopharmacology. (ed. Sirois, P.). Elsevier, Amsterdam. (in press).

SPREAFICO, F. and VECCHI, A. (1983) Immunomodulation by xenobiotics. The open field of immunotoxicology. In: Advances on Immunomodulators. (eds. Ambrogi, F. and Fudenberg, H.H.) Plenum Press, New York. (in press).

SPREAFICO, F., VECCHI, A., ANACLERIO, A., MORAS, M.L., TAGLIABUE, A., BARALE, C., MANTOVANI, A., SIRONI, M. and POLENTARUTTI, N. (1977) Experimental analysis of the effects of oral contraceptives on the function of the lymphoid system. p. 267. In: Pharmacology of Steroid Contraceptive Drugs. (eds. Garattini, S. and Berendes, H.W.) Raven Press, New York.

SPREAFICO, F., VECCHI, A., CONTI, G. and SIRONI, M. (1981a) On the heterogeneity of immunotherapeutic agents. p. 51. In: Advances in Immunopharmacology. (eds. Hadden, J., Chedid, L., Mullen, P. and Spreafico, F.) Pergamon Press, Oxford.

SPREAFICO, F., VECCHI, A., MANTOVANI, A., TAGLIABUE, A., SIRONI, M., LUINI, W. and GARATTINI, S. (1981b) The assessment of the immunotoxicity of xenobiotics. Experience with tetrachlorodibenzodioxin and saccharin. p. 295. In: Advances in Immunopharmacology. (eds. Hadden, J., Chedid, L., Mullen, P. and Spreafico, F.) Pergamon Press, Oxford.

VECCHI, A., MANTOVANI, A., SIRONI, M., LUINI, W., SPREAFICO, F. and GARATTINI, S. (1980) The effect of acute administration of 2,3,7,8-tetrachlorodibenzo-p-dioxin (TCDD) on humoral antibody production and cell-mediated activities in mice. Arch. Toxicol. Suppl. 4, 163.

VECCHI, A., SIRONI, M., CANEGRATI, M.A. and GARATTINI, S. (1983) Comparison of the immunosuppressive effects in mice of 2,3,7,8-tetrachlorodibenzo-p-dioxin (TCDD) and 2,3,7,8-tetrachlorodibenzofuran (TCDF). In: Chlorinated Dioxins and Dibenzofurans in the Total Environment. (eds. Keith, L.H., Choudhary, G. and Rappe, C.) Ann Arbor Science, Ann Arbor. (in press).

VECCHI, A., TAGLIABUE, A., MANTOVANI, A., ANACLERIO, A., BARALE, C. and SPREAFICO, F. (1976) Steroid contraceptive agents and immunological reactivity in experimental animals. Biomedicine 24, 231.

VOS, J.G., FAITH, R.E. and LUSTER, M.I. (1980) Immune alterations. p. 241. In: Halogenated Biphenyls, Terphenyls, Naphthalenes, Dibenzodioxins and Related Products. (ed. Kimbrough, R.D.) Elsevier, Amsterdam.

VOS, J.G. and MOORE, J.A. (1974) Suppression of cellular immunity in rats and mice by maternal treatment with 2,3,7,8-tetrachlorodibenzo-p-dioxin. Int. Arch. Allergy Appl. Immunol. 47, 777.

WALKER, W.S. (1976) Functional heterogeneity of macrophages. p. 91. In: Immunobiology of the Macrophage. (ed. Nelson, D.S.) Academic Press, London.

BENZENE-INDUCED IMMUNOTOXICITY: THE LYMPHOCYTE AS A TOOL FOR STUDYING SUBCELLULAR MECHANISMS OF TOXICITY

Richard D. Irons and Richard W. Pfeifer
Department of Pathology
Chemical Industry Institute of Toxicology
Research Triangle Park, NC, 27709, USA

From the perspective of an immunotoxicologist, the effects of chemicals on lymphocyte function are of interest because of the cell's pivotal role in immune responses. Apart from its significance as a target cell for immunotoxic agents, the lymphocyte also represents a powerful tool which can be used to study basic subcellular mechanisms of toxicity. In addition to the relatively obvious advantages of accessibility and sensitivity to various agents, the lymphocyte possesses a number of characteristics that make it an appropriate model for studying the effects of agents on cell growth and differentiation.

Nowell first discovered that phytohemagglutinin (PHA), a plant lectin isolated from the red kidney bean, will stimulate a proportion of normal lymphocytes to undergo blast transformation and division in culture (Nowell, 1960). Subsequently a large number of compounds have been identified that will stimulate lymphocyte proliferation _in vitro_. Lectins, in particular, are useful because they bind to saccharide groups on the lymphocyte plasma membrane and trigger a class or group of lymphocytes expressing particular saccharide moieties on their surface and therefore tend to bypass the rigid specificity demonstrated by lymphocytes toward antigens. The term, mitogen, is often used to describe a substance, lectin or not, that will induce DNA synthesis and division in normal lymphocytes.

The initial triggering event in mitogenesis appears to be confined to the cell surface membrane (Edelman, 1973). Mitogen stimulation therefore provides a tool for studying the transmission of messages from the cell surface to its interior and the regulation of subsequent cellular response. Lectin induced blastogenesis is dependent on cell-cell interaction. For example, the density of cells in culture will influence blastogenic response to lectin stimulation. This is important as a model for studying cell-cell communication and also in the context of examining lymphocyte interaction with non-lymphoid accessory cells, the macrophages and dendritic cells, which have been implicated in augmenting mitogen response. The precise sequence of events that lead to blastogenesis following lectin binding is unknown, nevertheless, the study of

NATO ASI Series, Vol. G2
Immunotoxicology. Edited by P. W. Mullen

these processes has led to the realization that cell growth response and cell-cell recognition are controlled through an assembly of interacting structures at or near the cell surface. Microfilaments (MF), microtubules (MT) and glycoprotein surface receptors have been postulated to form a surface modulating assembly that governs lectin-induced blastogenesis and receptor movement at the cell surface (Edelman, 1976; McClain, D'Eustachio and Edelman, 1977; McClain and Edelman, 1980). Microtubules, and microfilaments are referred to collectively as the cytoskeleton.

Microtubule disrupting agents that readily penetrate the cell disrupt normal blastogenic responses often in a biphasic manner, enhancing density-dependent lectin response at low concentrations and suppressing or inhibiting blastogenic response at higher concentrations (Edelman, 1976; Sherline and Mundy, 1977; Wang, Gunther and Edelman, 1975; Yoshinaga, Yoshinaga and Waksman, 1972; Himes and Houston, 1978; Elferink and Riemsera, 1980; Giordano and Lichtman, 1973; Irons, Neptun and Pfeifer, 1981). It should be emphasized that these events relate to a requirement for MT in G_0/G_1 events distinct from the well known requirement for MT integrity in spindle formation prior to mitosis. Furthermore, these effects do not involve changes in lectin binding and occur at concentrations of MT disrupting agents that do not result in cell death or interfere with energy production within the cell (Irons et al, 1981; Chaplin and Wedner, 1978; Lagunoff and Wan, 1979; Greene, Parker and Parker, 1976).

The cytoskeleton is also important in the regulation of cell surface receptor mobility and movement. In the free state, cell surface antigens are randomly distributed. The binding of a cross-linking ligand induces a clustering or patching of cell surface antigen through a passive process that requires neither active cell metabolism or viability. Patching is followed by a coalescense of bound surface antigen to form a cap at one end of the cell (capping). In contrast to patching, capping is energy dependent and requires MF integrity. Inhibitors of MF function will inhibit capping as will energy inhibitors or certain polyvalent ligands in very high concentrations such as concanavalin A (Con A) (Loor, 1977). Con A inhibition of capping is thought to be brought about through extensive cross linking of Con A surface receptors, restricting the movement of a wide range of receptors. Microtubules are involved in surface antigen restriction. Microtubule disrupting agents actually facilitate capping even in the presence of high concentrations of Con A (Loor, 1977). The relationship between surface receptor movement and blastogenesis is complex and incompletely understood, although it is evident that the two processes are linked. Experiments have demonstrated, for example, that Con A inhibition of capping will not block transmission of the mitogenic signal but will prevent blastogenic responses(McClain and Edelman, 1976).

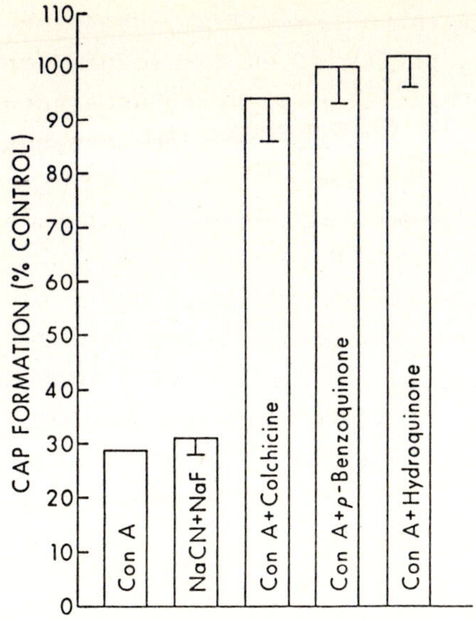

Figure 1 Facilitation of capping by microtubule inhibitors. Human peripheral lymphocytes were isolated as described for rat spleen cells (Irons et al, 1981). Cells were incubated at room temperature in the presence of 10^{-5} M HQ, p-BQ, 2.5 x 10^{-6} M colchicine, 100 mM NaCN/10 mM NaF, or phosphate buffered saline (control) for 10 min, followed by 15 min incubation with Con A (100 µg/ml). Capping was induced by incubation with fluorescein conjugated goat anti-human Ig (TAGO 1230), diluted 1/10, for 30 min at 37°C. Cells were examined using fluorescence microscopy and the number of caps/100 fluorescent cells determined. Values represent the mean ± 1 S.D. for three experiments.

Taken collectively, these phenomena provide us with a means of examining the effects of certain agents on cytoskeletal dependent processes within the cell. Benzene is probably the most widely recognized industrial chemical associated with toxicity to the blood and blood forming organs. Lymphocytes have been demonstrated to be among the most sensitive cells following exposure to benzene in vivo (Goldwater, 1941; Irons, Heck, Moore and Muirhead, 1979). Short term benzene exposure inhibits both T and B lymphocyte function and inhibits the ability of antigen reactive precursor B cells to generate antibody against a T-dependent antigen. Because of the indirect evidence associating the benzene metabolite, hydroquinone (HQ), with benzene toxicity (Weirda, Irons and Greenlee, 1981; Rickert, Edgar, Bus, Barrow and Irons, 1979; Irons, Dent, Baker, and Rickert, 1980; Greenlee and Irons, 1981; Greenlee, Gross and Irons, 1981), we examined the ability of HQ to produce immune suppression in mice after in vivo administration. HQ reduces both the frequency of immature B-cells and B- and T- cell mitogen response in spleen (Weirda and Irons, 1982).

Hydroquinone autoxidizes under physiologic conditions to form p-benzoquinone (p-BQ) (Irons, Greenlee, Wierda and Bus, 1982). In vitro studies reveal that HQ, and its oxidation product, p-benzoquinone, inhibit PHA mitogen response in culture in a bi-phasic manner similar to known MT disruptive agents. Furthermore, suppression occurs at concentrations of these metabolites that did not produce cell death or inhibit energy production within the cell. Catechol, a benzene metabolite that does not autoxodize to form its respective quinone, does not effectively suppress blastogenesis in vitro.

Microtubule assembly is sulfhydryl-dependent, and a number of sulfhydryl reagents are potent inhibitors of microtubule assembly. Sulfhydryl reagents which penetrate the cell disrupt cytoskeletal-dependent processes including blastogenesis. The sulfhydryl reactivity of benzoquinone is well known and led us to examine the possibility that the quinones altered lymphocyte function via a sulfhydryl-dependent disruption of MT assembly.

p-Benzoquinone is approximately twice as potent as HQ in suppressing PHA induced lymphocyte blastogenesis in culture which is consistent with the interpretation that p-BQ is the active form. The concentration range for suppression is approximately the same as observed for the cell-penetrating sulfhydryl reagents, NEM and cytochalasin A. Concentration

Table I. Effect of Hydroquinone, p-Benzoquinone and N-ethylmaleimide on PHA mitogen response in Ficoll-purified rat spleen cells.*

Concentration (M)	Treatment		
	Hydroquinone	p-Benzoquinone	N-ethylmaleimide
1×10^{-4}	0	0	0.5
1×10^{-5}	2	1	1
1×10^{-6}	136	44	77
8×10^{-7}	156	38	-
6×10^{-7}	190	72	-
4×10^{-7}	207	75	-

* Values are expressed as percent of control. Spleen cell isolation and culture conditions were the same as published previously (Irons et al, 1981).

dependent protection against suppression of blastogenesis by any of these agents is achieved only in the presence of sulfhydryl compounds such as cysteine or dithiothreitol. That these events involve intracellular SH groups critical for blastogenesis is evident in that 5,5'-dithiobis(2-nitrobenzoic acid) (DTNB), a poorly penetrating sulfhydryl reagent, has no demonstrable effect on blastogenesis (Irons et al, 1981).

At low concentrations p-benzoquinone and HQ appear to selectively interfere with MT-dependent functions. Both will effectively facilitate ligand-induced lymphocyte capping in the presence of inhibitory concentrations of con A, confirming that energy metabolism and MF integrity are preserved at concentrations of these agents that interfere with MT function. Finally, HQ and p-BQ inhibit MT assembly directly *in vitro*.

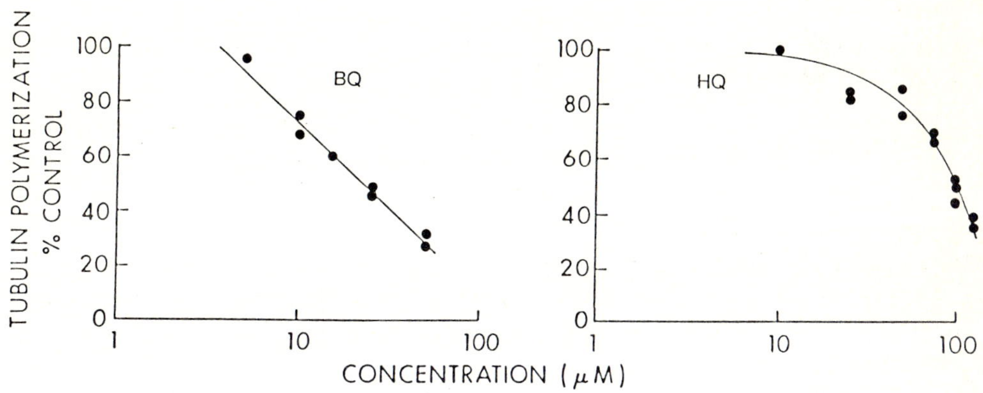

Figure 2 Inhibition of microtubule assembly by p-benzoquinone and hydroquinone *in vitro*. Tubulin isolation and experimental conditions have previously been described (Irons et al, 1981).

Although the role of the cytoskeleton in normal cell function is complex and incompletely understood, it appears to be intimately involved in regulating the cell's response to events occurring at its surface. Microtubules appear to constitute a particularly sensitive sulfhydryl-dependent target, important to normal growth control of the mammalian cell which are uniquely sensitive to cell penetrating sulfhydryl alkylating reagents such as quinones. The use of lymphocyte culture systems in combination with biochemical methods provides a means to distinguish between agents with predominantly cytoskeletal reactivity and those producing additional effects at the same concentrations and constitutes a powerful tool for studying cell growth regulation and cell-cell communication.

REFERENCES

CHAPLIN, D.D. and WEDNER, H.J. (1978) Inhibition of lectin-induced lymphocyte activation of diamide and other sulfhydryl reagents. Cell. Immunol. 36, 303.

EDELMAN, G.M. (1973) In: Control of Proliferation in Animal Cells Cold Spring Harbor Laboratories, NY, p. 357.

EDELMAN, G.M. (1976) Surface modulation in cell recognition and cell growth. Science 192, 218.

ELFERINK, J.G.R. and RIEMSERA, J.C. (1980) Effects of sulfhydryl reagents on phagocytosis and exocytosis in rabbit polymorphonuclear leukocytes. Chem. Biol. Interact. 30, 139.

GIORDANO, G.I. and LICHTMAN, M.A. (1973) The role of sulfhydryl groups in human neutrophil adhesion, movement and particle ingestion. J. Cell Physiol. 82, 387.

GOLDWATER, L.J. (1941) Disturbances in the blood following exposure to benzol. J. Lab. Clin. Med. 26, 957.

GREENE, W.C., PARKER, C.M. and PARKER, C.W. (1976) Colchicine-sensitive structures and lymphocyte activation. J. Immunol. 117, 1015.

GREENLEE, W.F., GROSS, E.A. and IRONS, R.D. (1981) Relationship between benzene toxicity and the disposition of ^{14}C-labelled bengene metabolites in the rat. Chem. Biol. Interact. 33, 285.

GREENLEE, W.F. and IRONS, R.D. (1981) Modulation of benzene-induced lymphocytopenia in the rat by 2,4,5, 2',4',5'-hexachlorobiphenyl and 3,4,3'4'-tetrachlorobiphenyl. Chem. Biol. Interact. 33, 345.

HIMES, R.H. and HOUSTON, L.L. (1976) The action of cytochalasin A on the in vitro polymerization of brain tubulin and muscle G-actin. J. Supramol. Struct. 5, 81.

IRONS, R.D., DENT, J.G., BAKER, T.S. and RICKERT, D.E. (1980) Benzene is metabolized and covalently bound in bone marrow in situ. Chem. Biol. Interact. 30, 241.

IRONS, R.D., GREENLEE, W.F., WIERDA, D. and BUS, J.S. (1982) In: Biological Reactive Intermediates II. (eds. Snyder, R., Parke, D.V., Kocsis, J.J., Jollow, D.J., Gibson, G.G. and Witmer, C.M.) Plenum Press, NY and London, p. 229.

IRONS, R.D., HECK, H. d'A., MOORE, B.J. and MUIRHEAD, K.A. (1979) Effects of short-term benzene administration on bone marrow cell cycle kinetics in the rat. Toxicol. Appl. Pharmacol. 51, 399.

IRONS, R.D., NEPTUN, D.A. and PFEIFER, R.W. (1981) Inhibition of lymphocyte transformation and microtubule assembly by quinone metabolites of benzene: Evidence for a common mechanism. J. Reticuloendothelial Soc. 30, 359.

LAGUNOFF, D. and WAN, H. (1979) Inhibition of histamine release from rat mast cells by cytochalasin A and other sulfhydryl reagents. Biochem. Pharmacol. 28, 1765.

LOOR, F. (1977) Structure and dynamics of the lymphocyte surface in relation to differentiation, recognition and activation. Prog. Allergy 23, 1.

McCLAIN, D.L., D'EUSTACHIO, P. and EDELMAN, G.M. (1977) Role of surface modulating assemblies in growth control of normal and transformed fibroblasts. Proc. Natl. Acad. Sci. U.S.A. 74, 666.

McCLAIN, D.L. and EDELMAN, G.M. (1976) Analysis of the stimulation-inhibition paradox exhibited by lymphocytes exposed to concanavalin A. J. Exp. Med. 144, 1494.

McCLAIN, D.L. and EDELMAN, G.M. (1980) Density dependent stimulation and inhibition of cell growth by agents that disrupt microtubules. Proc. Natl. Acad. Sci. U.S.A. 77, 2748.

NOWELL, P.C. (1960) Phytohemagglutinin: An initiator of mitosis in cultures of normal human leukocytes. Cancer Res. 20, 462.

RICKERT, D.E., EDGAR, T.S., BUS, J.S., BARROW, C.S. and IRONS, R.D. (1979) Benzene disposition in the rat after exposure by inhalation. Toxicol. Appl. Pharmacol. 49, 417.

SHERLINE, P. and MUNDY, G.R. (1977) Role of the tubulin-microtubule system in lymphocyte activation. J. Cell Biol. 74, 371.

WANG, J.L., GUNTHER, G.R. and EDELMAN, G.M. (1975) Inhibition by colchicine of the mitogenic stimulation of lymphocytes prior to the S phase. J. Cell Biol. 66, 128.

WIERDA, D. and IRONS, R.D. (1982) Hydroquinone and catechol reduce the frequency of progenitor B lymphocytes in mouse spleen and bone marrow. Immunopharmacol. 4, 41.

WIERDA, D., IRONS, R.D. and GREENLEE, W.F. (1981) Immunotoxicity in C57BL/6 mice exposed to benzene and aroclor 1254. Toxicol. Appl. Pharmacol. 60, 410.

YOSHINAGA, M., YOSHINAGA, A. and WAKSMAN, B.H. (1972) Recognition of lymphocyte response in vitro; potentiation and inhibition of rat lymphocyte responses to antigens and mitogens by cytochalasin B. Proc. Natl. Acad. Sci. U.S.A. 69, 3251

ENVIRONMENTAL ESTROGENS AND THEIR EFFECT ON IMMUNE RESPONSES

Michael I. Luster[1], Gary A. Boorman[1], Howard T. Hayes[1], Jack H. Dean[2], Lily Hong[1], Richard Pfeifer[1], Kenneth S. Korach[1] and Linda Rhodes[1]

[1]National Institute of Environmental Health Sciences
P.O. Box 12233
Research Triangle Park, NC 27709, U.S.A.

[2]Chemical Industry Institute of Toxicology
P.O. Box 12137
Research Triangle Park, NC 27709, U.S.A.

In mice administration of pharmacological levels of estrogens causes a rapid but not necessarily irreversible atrophy of the thymus (reviewed by Dougherty, 1952). From numerous studies, it is apparent that sex steroids influence lymphoid development, particularly the thymus although the mechanisms are not understood (Sobhon and Jirasatthan, 1974). Similarly, evidence exists that the thymus plays a role in the female sexual maturation, at least in perinatal life (Besedovsky and Sorkin, 1974). Even physiological levels of estrogen (i.e. 17β-estradiol and estrone) are capable of modulating immune responses. This is evidenced by the observation that female mice have superior humoral immunity (HMI) and somewhat inferior cell mediated immunity (CMI) as compared to age matched males and these differences can be negated by castration (reviewed by Ahlquist, 1976). The effects of supraphysiological levels of estrogen on immune processes are multi-fold. Exogenous estrogens are a recognized stimulant of the reticuloendothelial system (RES) which increases splenic and hepatic phagocytic activity (reviewed by Vernon-Roberts, 1969). Estradiol alters antibody regulation and has been associated with the development of autoimmune disease in mice (Roubinian, Papoian and Tolal, 1977). Treatment with higher levels of exogenous estrogens inhibit cellular immune functions (reviewed by Ahlquist, 1976).

ENVIRONMENTAL ESTROGENS

Of interest to toxicologists is the fact that many xenobiotics, natural products and potential environmental pollutants possess estrogenic activity and demonstrate high binding affinity to the cytosolic and nuclear estrogen receptors (reviewed by Katzenellenbogen, Katzenellenbogen, Tatee, Robertson and Landvatter, 1980). While many of these chemicals are only weakly estrogenic, it is becoming apparent that either chronic exposure or acute exposure to weakly estrogenic compounds which

NATO ASI Series, Vol. G2
Immunotoxicology. Edited by P. W. Mullen

are not readily excreted (e.g. kepone) may lead to abnormal reproductive development and potential neoplasia (reviewed by Eroschenko and Palmiter, 1980). Several xenobiotics shown to have estrogenic activity include o,p'-DDT, methoxychlor and chlordecone. Some natural products that demonstrate binding affinity for the estrogen receptor are the flavones genistin, mirestrol and the fluorescent coumestrol. The mycotoxin zearalanone (P-1502) and its more potent metabolite zearalanol (P-1496) produced from the fungus Fusarium also show remarkable binding affinity for the receptor.

Diethylstilbestrol (DES) is a nonsteroidal synthetic compound with similar uterotrophic potency and binding activity in mice as 17β-estradiol (Korach, Metzler and McLachlan, 1978). The compound has been extensively employed as a therapeutic agent in humans as estrogen replacement, in prostate cancer therapy and as a component of contraceptive medication. There is a large amount of evidence, however, that DES may be potentially carcinogenic in humans and laboratory animals and has been associated with endometrial cancer, breast cancer, and vaginal adenocarcinoma (reviewed in McLachlan, 1980). In female mice, DES suppresses specific immunity following either prenatal (Luster, Faith, McLachlan and Clark, 1979), postnatal (Kalland, 1980a), or adult (Sljivic and Warr, 1973; Luster, Boorman, Dean, Luebke and Lawson, 1980) exposure. In addition, both estradiol (Seaman, Gindhart, Greenspan, Blackman and Talae, 1979) and DES (Kalland, 1980b) depresses natural killer cell activity, induces bone marrow myelotoxicity (Boorman, Luster, Dean and Wilson, 1980) and induces inflammatory macrophages (Boorman, et al, 1980). DES also alters host resistance to agents that are dependent upon normal T-cells and macrophage functions. Increased susceptibility has been reported following challenge with Listeria monocytogenes or Trichinella spiralis and increased tumor development occurred following challenge with syngeneic tumor cells in DES treated mice (Dean, Luster, Boorman, Luebke and Lauer, 1980). Resistance to infectious agents which are primarily dependent upon B-cell processes (e.g. Plasmodium) are not readily effected by DES exposure (unpublished data). It has not been determined whether this immunologic dysfunction serves directly as an adduct in the development of neoplasia.

Zearalanol (P-1496) is an estrogenic metabolite of the mycotoxin zearalanone which is produced by various species of Fusarium. It possesses approximately 17% of the binding affinity of 17β-estradiol but less than 1% of its uterotrophic activity (Katzenellenbogen, Katzenellenbogen and Mordecai, 1979). P-1496 has been proposed to be used as a growth promotant in sheep and cattle and was of interest to study immunologically for a number of reasons. First, as seen in Figure 1, it is structurally similar to DES and estradiol since it contains a phenolic ring structure similar to the "A ring region" of estradiol (reviewed by Pathre and Mirocha, 1980). The phenolic ring structure is believed responsible for the receptor binding affinity and specificity of estrogenic compounds. Secondly, while zearalanol is weakly estrogenic in the uterus, it readily reacts with the avid liver estrogen receptor (Powell-Jones, Raeford and Lucier, 1981). Thus, it was felt that P-1496 may help in distinguishing the divergent effects observed with DES on the immune system, i.e. suppressed CMI and activated macrophages as well as eludicating the relationship, if any, between uterotrophic activity and estrogen-induced immunodeficiency.

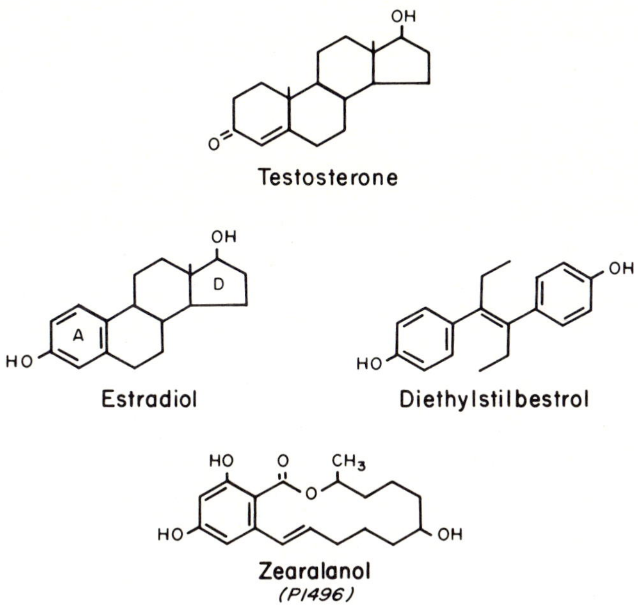

Figure 1 Structural formulae of testosterone, DES, zearalanol and estradiol.

EXPERIMENTAL RESULTS

Macrophage function was evaluated by the growth inhibition assay employing plastic adherent resident peritoneal cells. This assay determines the ability of macrophages to inhibit the in vitro growth of MBL-2 leukemia target cells and is a measure of inflammatory macrophages (Dean, Padarathsingh and Keys, 1978). In some cases macrophage activity was also examined by determining the percent of resident peritoneal cells capable of phagocytizing fluorescent beads. The data in Table I demonstrate that macrophages from mice exposed to equimolar concentrations of DES, 17β-estradiol or P-1496 quantitatively induce a similar degree of macrophage activation as determined by the growth inhibition assay. In contrast, testosterone and its more active metabolite 5α-dihydrotestosterone (Bruchovsky and Wilson, 1968) did not effect macrophage function. Testosterone and 5α-dihydrotestosterone which possess some estrogenic activity (Schmidt and Katzenellenbogan, 1979) were of interest to study because they are structurally similar to estradiol in the "D-ring region", but not "A-ring region" of the molecule.

Table I. Tumor cell cytostatic activity of adherent resident peritoneal macrophages in female mice administered estrogenic compounds.

Treatment[a]	^{3}H-TdR Incorp. in MBL-2 Target Cells (CPM ± SEM x 10^{-3})	Percent Cytostasis
Corn oil	75 ± 4[b]	-
DES	29 ± 7*	62%
17β-Estradiol	30 ± 3*	60%
P-1496	34 ± 6*	54%
Testosterone	90 ± 7	38%↑
5α-Dihydrotestosterone	74 ± 3	1%

[a]Adult female mice were administered equimolar concentrations (2.8 μmoles/mouse) subcutaneous in corn oil over a 5 day period.

[b]Values were obtained at 20:1 macrophage to MBL-2 target cell ratio. Since control values are subject to slight daily variation, data in Tables I and II are relative to control for that particular day.

*$p < 0.01$ vs controls.

The effects of estrogens on specific immune function were evaluated by examining delayed hypersensitivity, antibody plaque forming cells and splenic lymphocyte blastogenic responses. Table II summarizes some of these results in which lymphoproliferative response to mitogens and allogencic leukocytes were determined. DES and 17β-estradiol severely depressed the T-cell response to mitogen (PHA) as well as allogeneic leukocyte in the mixed leukocyte culture response (MLC) but unlike macrophage function, P-1496 did not alter lymphoblastogenic responses. A slight, but significant suppression also occurred in mice treated with 5α-dihydrotestosterone. The B-cell response following stimulation with lipopolysaccharide was essentially unaltered in estrogen treated mice, however, suppression occurred in 5α-dihydrotesterone treated mice which probably reflects an androgen effect. In this respect earlier studies revealed that testosterone primarily acted on the B-lymphocyte population (Fujii, Nawa, Tsuchiya, Matsuno, Fukumoto, Fukuda and Kotani, 1975). Thymus atrophy occurred in almost all treated mice but was most evident in DES and 17β-estradiol treated groups and correlated with depression of T-cell blastogenic responses. Histologically, the thymus atrophy was characterized by severe depletion of cortical lymphocytes.

Table II Thymic atrophy and lymphoblastogenic responses in adult female mice treated with various compounds.

Treatment[a]	Thymic Atrophy (% change)	^{3}H-TdR Incorp. (nCPM x 10^{-3})[b] (% change)		
		PHA	LPS	MLC
Corn oil	-	34 ± 2	22 ± 3	38 ± 5
DES	79↓**	20 ± 1** (41↓)	25 ± 3 (14↑)	13 ± 3** (66↓)
17β-Estradiol	75↓**	23 ± 3** (32↓)	30 ± 4* (34↑)	20 ± 2** (47↓)
17β-Estradiol (10X)	ND	15 ± 1** (56↑)	23 ± 2 (4↑)	ND
P-1496	25↓*	33 ± 2 (3↓)	24 ± 2 (9↑)	34 ± 6 (11↓)
Testosterone	14↓	34 ± 3 (0)	16 ± 4 (27↓)	34 ± 3
5α-Dihydrotestosterone	46↓**	27 ± 2* (21↓)	11 ± 2* (50↓)	44 ± 5

[a]Adult female mice were administered equimolar concentrations (2.8μmoles/mouse) subcutaneously in corn oil over a 5 day period.

[b]Mean ± SEM of 7 mice/group. Data are expressed as net CPM = counts per minute (CPM) in stimulated cultures - CPM in cultures without stimulator.

*$p < 0.05$ vs controls. ** $p < 0.01$ vs controls. ND = not done.

In order to insure that the selective effect by P-1496 on macrophage activity was specific and not simply due to differences in response time between estrogen-induced macrophage and lymphocyte dysfunction, it was necessary to perform kinetic studies. Increased macrophage activity, as determined in vitro by the MBL-2 growth inhibition assay, was observed in mice from days 3 to 6 following a single exposure to either P-1496 or estradiol (data not shown). Similarly, lymphocyte function as assessed in vitro by PHA responsiveness was significantly depressed in mice from days 3 to 5 following an acute exposure to 17β-estradiol. This suggested that the immunoregulatory disassociation with these compounds was specific and not dependent upon time of response.

Studies by Stimson and Hunter (1980) suggested that some immunotoxicity induced by estrogens are mediated through the thymus following estrogen treatment. This was suggested by the fact that sera from estrogen treated rats, but not estrogen exposed thymectomized (Tx) rats were capable of affecting several in vitro correlates of immune function. In experiments performed in our laboratory, adult female mice were surgically Tx, subsequently exposed to DES or 17β-estradiol and examined immunologically (Table III). Unlike non-Tx estrogen treated mice, inflammatory macrophages were not induced in thymectomized estrogen exposed mice. In contrast to macrophage activity, it appeared that pre-Tx failed to inhibit estrogen-induced immunosuppression of lymphocyte function as determined by the MLC response. The PHA response in non-estrogen treated controls was significantly depressed as a result of Tx complicating interpretation of mitogen responses. In data not shown, estrogen-induced inhibition of bone marrow porligerative responses (i.e. CFU-S and CFU-GM) were also prevented by pre-Tx.

Table III Effect of adult thymectomy on estrogen-induced immune alterations.

Parameter	Non-thymectomized			Thymectomized		
	Control	DES	Estradiol	Control	DES	Estradiol
MACROPHAGE FUNCTION						
Percent Cell Phagocytizing	20	47** (135↑)	47** (135↑)	24 (16↑)	31 (55↑)	29 (45↑)
Cytostasis (^{3}H-TdR[b] Incorp. x 10^{-3})	58	30** (48↓)	36** (38↓)	45 (6↓)	68 (15↑)	76** (31↑)
LYMPHOBLASTOGENESIS (^{3}H-TdR Incorp.; nCPM x 10^{-3})						
MLC	19±5	6±1** (68↓)	10±1** (47↓)	15±1 (21↓)	5±1** (74↓)	7±1** (63↓)
PHA	25±2	12±2* (52↓)	16±1** (36↓)	11±1** (56↓)	8±1** (68↓)	12±3** (52↓)

[a]Mice were surgically Tx and treated with either DES (4.0 mg/kg) or estradiol (16 mg/kg) two days later for 5 consecutive days. Three days following the last treatment animals were tested. Percent change from non-Tx controls in parenthesis below.

[b]Represents mean of two replicates.

** $p < 0.01$ vs controls.

These data demonstrate that many of the immunomodulatory effects induced by estrogens appear to be related to the thymus. Although the manifestations of the estrogen/thymus interplay is obviously complex and is probably not responsible for CMI suppression, it is interesting to note that we saw a similar biomodal disassociation of immune effects in mice exposed to P-1496. That is, P-1496 exposure altered macrophage activity and bone marrow function without affecting lymphocyte blastogenesis. The molecular events associated with these interactions are unknown but are of particular interest because the immunological manifestations are preceded by thymic atrophy. This study is also of interest in another respect, in that it provides further evidence that thymic regulation of immune responses are not restricted to perinatal life as has been generally thought.

Estrogenic activity in various target organs (e.g. uterus, anterior pituitary/hypothalmus) are mediated through a cytosolic receptor (Korach and Muldoon, 1974). Estrogen enters the cell where binding occurs to a specific intracellular receptor. This receptor-ligand complex undergoes a conformational change, enters the nucleus and is believed to interact with chromatin to stimulate gene expression. In this respect, estrogen receptor binding activity has been reported in the rat thymus cytosol (Gillette and Gillette, 1979). In studies performed in our laboratory, estrogen receptors with relatively high binding affinities were identified in mouse thymus (prepared from adult female mice) but not in the adherent cell population or in gradient purified splenic lymphocytes suggesting their presence in thymic epithelium. This would indirectly suggest that the immunomodulatory effects associated with estrogens are mediated indirectly through the thymus.

To further examine the possibility that estrogen-induced immunodeficiency is mediated through a receptor mechanism, we have examined the activity of several estrogen antagonists. Two groups of antiestrogens have been identified and include derivatives of triphenylethylene and derivatives of diphenyl (dihydro- or tetrahydro-) naphthalene, the most notable being Tamoxifen and Nofoxidine, respectively (reviewed by Sutherland and Murphy, 1982). If one assumes that estrogen-mediated immunomodulation is mediated through interaction with a receptor, then <u>in vivo</u> administration with DES or estradiol concurrently with an estrogen antagonist should mitigate some of these effects. As can be seen in Table IV, administration of Tamoxifen simultaneously with estrogens prevents estrogen-induced suppression of pleuripotent stem cell proliferation (CFU-S) as well as splenic lymphoblastogenic responses (Nafoxidine data not shown). Estrogen-induced thymic atrophy was only partially prevented by the anti-estrogens.

Table IV The effects of estrogen antagonist on estrogen-induced immunomodulation.

Treatment	Thymic Atrophy (% Change)	Lymphoblastogenic PHA Responses (CPM x 10^{-3})	Stem Cell Proliferation (CFU-S/5 x 10^4 Cells)
Control	-	36 ± 4	16.8 ± 0.4
DES	59↓**	12 ± 2**	14.4 ± 0.1**
Tamoxifen	14↓	27 ± 1	16.7 ± 0.2
Tamoxifen + DES	39↓**	47 ± 3	16.2 ± 0.4

Adult female mice were administered 50 mg/kg of tamoxifen on day 1 and day 2 while appropriate mice received 16 mg/kg DES on day 2 only. Animals were sacrificed and tested on day 5.

CONCLUSIONS

In summary, administration of potent estrogens selectively affects immune responses. This immunologic profile is consistent with myelotoxicity, suppression of CMI and activation of macrophage function. Modulation of several of these parameters is mediated through the thymus since pre-thymectomy abolishes estrogen-induced macrophage activation and myelotoxicity but does not inhibit depression of CMI. These effects can also be disassociated chemically in that P-1496 is selective for macrophage activation while 5α-dihydrotestosterone apparently is selective for CMI. This may be due to structural differences since P-1496 is similar to DES and estradiol in the A-ring region while testosterone and dihydrotestosterone possesses D-ring region structural similarities. However, underlying this explanation is the demonstration that many of these effects may be mediated through an estrogen receptor mechanism as suggested by inhibition of these effects using estrogen antagonist and the presence of receptor in the thymus. Thus, many of these effects may depend upon relative receptor binding affinity of the compound which would mediate hormonal effects in lymphoid tissue.

REFERENCES

AHLQUIST, J. (1976) Endocrine influences on lymphatic organs, immune responses, inflammation and autoimmunity. Acta Endocrinologica (Supp. 206) 83, 1.

BESEDOVSKY, H.O. and SORKIN, E. (1974) Thymus involvement in female sexual maturation. Nature 249, 356.

BOORMAN, G.A., LUSTER, M.I., DEAN, J.H. and WILSON, R.E. (1980) The effect of adult exposure to diethylstilbestrol in the mouse on macrophage function. J. Reticulo. Soc. 28, 547.

BRUCHOVSKY, N. and WILSON, J.D. (1968) The intranuclear binding of testosterone and 5α-androstan 17βol-3one by rat prostate. J. Biol. Chem. 243, 5953.

DEAN, J.H., LUSTER, M.I., BOORMAN, G.A., LUEBKE, R.W. and LAUER, L.D. (1980) The effect of adult exposure to diethylstilbestrol in the mouse: Alterations in tumor susceptibility and host resistance parameters. J. Reticulo. Soc. 28, 571.

DEAN, J.H., PADARATHSINGH, M.L. and KEYS, L. (1978) Response of murine leukemia to combined BCNU-maleic anhydride-vinyl ether (MVC) adjuvant therapy and correlation with macrophage activation by MVC in the in vitro growth inhibition assay. Cancer Treat. Rep. 62, 1807.

DOUGHERTY, T.F. (1952) Effect of hormones on lymphatic tissue. Physiol. Rev. 32, 379.

EROSCHENKO, V.P. and PALMITER, R.D. (1980) Estrogenicity of ketone in birds and mammals. In Estrogens in the Environment, ed. McLachlan, J.A. (Elsevier, North Holland), pp. 305-325.

FUJII, H., NAWA, Y., TSUCHIYA, H., MATSUNO, K., FUKUMOTO, T., FUKUDA, S. and KOTANI, M. (1975) Effect of a single administration of testosterone on the immune response and lymphoid tissues in mice. Cell. Immunol. 20, 315.

GILLETTE, S. and GILLETTE, R.W. (1979) Changes in thymic estrogen receptor expression following orchidectomy. Cell. Immunol. 42, 194.

KALLAND, T. (1980a) Alterations of antibody response in female mice after neonatal exposure to diethylstilbestrol. J. Immunol. 124, 194.

KALLAND, T. (1980b) Reduced natural killer activity in female mice after neonatal exposure to diethylstilbestrol. J. Immunol. 124, 1297.

KATZENELLENBOGEN, B.S., KATZENELLENBOGEN, J.A. and MORDECAI, D. (1979) Zearalenones: Charactreization of the estrogenic potencies and receptor interactions of a series of fungal β-resorcyclic acid lactones. Endocrinology 105, 33.

KATZENELLENBOGEN, J.A., KATZENELLENBOGEN, B.S., TATEE, T., ROBERTSON, D.W. and LANDVATTER, S.W. (1980) In Estrogens in the Environment, ed. McLachlan, J.A. (Elsevier, North Holland), pp. 33-51.

KORACH, K.S., METZLER, M. and McLACHLAN, J.A. (1978) Estrogenic activity in vivo and in vitro of some diethylstilbestrol metabolites and analogs. Proc. Natl. Acad. Sci. 75, 468.

KORACH, K.S. and MULDOON, T.G. (1974) Characterization of the interaction between estradiol and its cytoplasmic receptor in the rat anterior pituitary gland. Biochemistry 13, 1932.

LUSTER, M.I., FAITH, R.E., McLACHLAN, J.A. and CLARK, G.C. (1979) Effect of in utero exposure to diethylstilbestrol on the immune response in mice. Toxicol. Appl. Pharmacol. 47, 287.

LUSTER, M.I., BOORMAN, G.A., DEAN, J.H., LUEBKE, R.W. and LAWSON, L.D. (1980) The effect of adult exposure to diethylstilbestrol in the mouse: Alterations in immunological function. J. Reticulo. Soc. 28, 561.

McLACHLAN, J.A. (1980) Estrogens in the Environment, Developments in Toxicology and Environmental Science, Vol. 5, (Elsevier, North Holland).

PATHRE, S.V. and MIROCHA, C.J. (1980) Mycotoxins as estrogens. In Estrogens in the Environment, ed. McLachlan, J.A. (Elsefier, North Holland), pp. 265-278.

POWELL-JONES, W., RAEFORD, S. and LUCIER, G.W. (1981) Binding properties of zearalenone mycotoxins to hepatic estrogen receptors. Molec. Pharmacol. 20, 35.

ROUBINIAN, J.R., PAPOIAN, R. and TOLAL, N. (1977) Androgenic hormones modulate autoantibody responses and improve survival in murine lupus. J. Clin, Invest. 59, 1066.

SCHMIDT, W.N. and KATZENELLENBOGEN, B.S. (1979) Androgen-uterine interactions: An assessment of androgen interaction with the testosterone and estrogen receptor systems and stimulation of uterine growth and progesterone-receptor synthesis. Mol. Cell Endocrinol. 15, 91.

SEAMAN, W.E., GINDHART, T.D., GREENSPAN, J.S., BLACKMAN, M. and TALAE,N. (1979) Natural killer cells, bone and the bone marrow: Studies in estrogen-treated mice and in congenitally osteopetrotic (mi/mi) mice. J. Immunol. 122, 2541.

SLIVIC, V.S. and WARR, G.W. (1973) Oestrogens and immunity. Period. Biol. 75, 231.

SOBHON, P. and JIRASATTHAN, C. (1974) Effect of sex hormones on the thymus and lymphoid tissues of ovariectomized rats. Acta. Anat. 89, 211.

STIMSON, W.H. and HUNTER, I.C. (1980) Oestrogen-induced immunoregulation mediated through the thymus. J. Clin. Lab. Immunol. 4, 27.

SUTHERLAND, R.L. and MURPHY, L.C. (1982) Mechanisms of oestrogen antagonism by nonsteroidal antioestrogens. Molec. Cellular Endocrin. 25, 5.

VERNON-ROBERTS, B. (1969) The effect of steroid hormones on macrophage activity. Int. Rev. Cytol. 25, 133.

IMMUNOSUPPRESSION BY THE TUMOR PROMOTING PHORBOL DIESTER TPA: A POSSIBLE EPIGENETIC MECHANISM IN CARCINOGENESIS

Jack H. Dean[1], Michael I Luster[2],
Edward C. Ward[1], and Lloyd D. Lauer[1]

[1]Chemical Industry Institute of Toxicology and
[2]National Institute of Environmental Health Sciences
Research Triangle Park, NC 27709, U.S.A.

The immune system is a complex network of interrelated lymphoid and myeloid cells which is primarily responsible for protection from infectious agents and responsible for rejection of allografts and neoplasms. Immunocompetence is best viewed as a continuous spectrum ranging from "normal" to severely impaired as is found in acquired or severe combined immunodeficiency diseases (e.g. •AIDS or SCID). Within this continuum are various degrees of immune dysfunction some of which are expressed as altered host resistance. For example, a slight suppression may lead to a prolongation of viral infections or the development of bacterial infections. Moderate suppression could lead to chronic or opportunistic infections or enhancement of tumor growth, while marked suppression may lead to lethal infections and death.

One proposed function of the immune system is that of immunosurveillance against arising neoplasms. The finding that many tumors express tumor specific antigens (TSA) (Prehn and Main, 1957; Old, Boyse, Clarke and Cresswell, 1962; Baldwin, 1973; Mastrangelo, Laucius and Outzen, 1974; Dean, McCoy, Lewis, Appella and Law, 1975) led to the hypothesis that the immune system recognizes these "foreign" antigens on arising tumors and eliminates them before they become established (Burnet, 1970). If the immune system was to become perturbed, such that it could no longer recognize the "neo"-antigens, or if non-antigenic tumors arose then progressive growth could occur. There is some experimental justification for this type of mechanism since spontaneously arising tumors are, in general, weakly antigenic (Klein and Klein, 1977a; Klein and Klein, 1977b). In addition, tumors which arise early after exposure to a carcinogen are generally more antigenic then those which arise after a long latency period possibly indicating that the immune system has been able to select for less antigenic variants among the transformed phenotypes

NATO ASI Series, Vol. G2
Immunotoxicology. Edited by P. W. Mullen

(Prehn, 1963; Sjogren, 1965). Further evidence for the role of the immune system in the resistance against arising neoplasms comes from studies on immunocompromised hosts (for review see Penn, 1982). For example, the overall incidence of de novo cancer among organ transplant recipients undergoing immunosuppressive therapy to prevent allograft rejection has been found to be unusually high. In a 10 year study of kidney transplant recipients the cancer incidence ranged from 26 to 47% (Sheil, Mahony, Horvath, Johnson, Teller, Stewart and May, 1981).

It was originally believed that the primary mechanism of tumor resistance operated via cell-mediated immune responses(CMI), involving predominantly cytotoxic T-cells against "neo"-antigens thought to be expressed on the tumors (Baldwin, 1973; Klein, 1966). Recently, another lymphoid cell has been identified which is also thought to play a central role in the immunological resistance against neoplasms, the natural killer (NK) cell (for review see Herberman, Djeu, Kay, et al, 1979). The NK cell is thought to be a lymphocyte which may share parentage with both monocytes and T-cells (Herberman and Ortaldo, 1981). NK cells possess the ability to distinguish between normal and transformed cells in vitro and to selectively kill those cells which are transformed (for review see Kiessling and Wigżell, 1979). Evidence for the in vivo functioning of NK cells in immune surveillance against tumors comes from studies with nude mice. Nude mice are deficient in functional T-cells yet they do not exhibit an increased incidence of spontaneous or chemically induced tumors (Outzen and Custer, 1975; Stutman, 1978; Kripke and Borsos, 1974) and indeed are more resistant to tumor transplants than normal controls (Warner, Woodruff and Burton, 1977; Greenberg and Greene, 1976). Subsequent studies revealed that nude mice have an increased level of natural killer cells compared to conventional mice and often can reject tumor transplants better than normal mice (Warner, et al, 1977). Beige mice, which have a mutation resulting in depressed NK activity while retaining many of their CMI parameters (Roder and Duwe, 1979), develop tumors more rapidly and at a higher frequency than normal mice upon challenge with transplantable tumors (Talmadge, Meyers, Prieur and Starkey, 1980a; Talmadge, Meyers, Prieur and Starkey, 1980b; Karre, Klein, Kiessling, Klein and Roder, 1980). NK cells have also been implicated in the metastatic process since some tumor sublines which are more sensitive to NK-mediated lysis have been found to be less metastatic than NK resistant sublines (Kawase, Urdal, Brooks and Henney, 1982). These studies, taken together with the studies on cell-mediated immunity, indicate that thymus-dependent lymphocytes and NK cells are active in immunosurveillance against arising tumors.

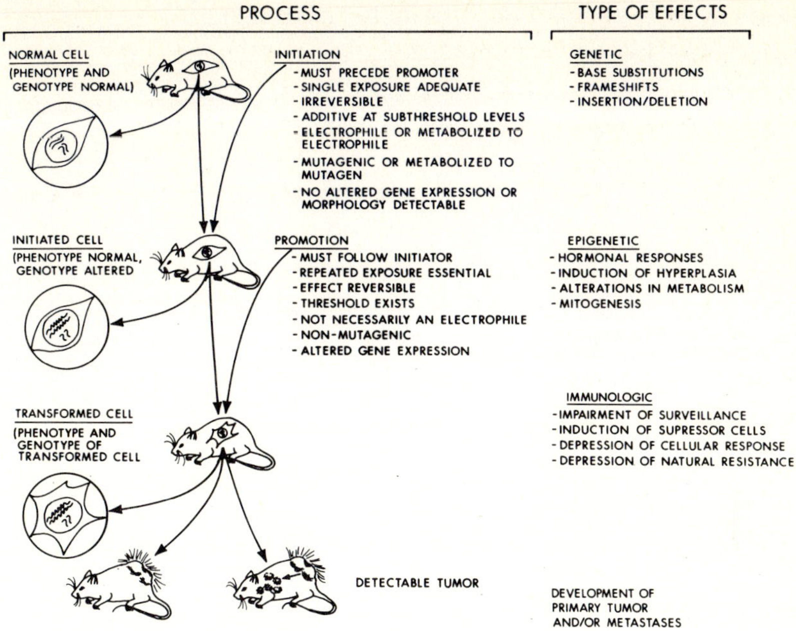

Figure 1 Diagramatic sketch of two stage tumor promotion model showing points where immune alteration may potentiate tumor development.

The role of the immune response in the development of carcinogen induced tumors is complex and ill-defined. However, immunosuppression has been shown to increase the incidence of tumors in carcinogen treated mice (Stjensward, 1966; Outzen, 1980). Figure 1 is a diagramatic representation of the two step mechanism of carcinogenesis (Bernblum, 1975) illustrating where we believe a depression of the immune system may allow for tumor expression. Cells which have been initiated are thought to display the phenotype of the normal cell while the genotype has been altered to that of the transformed cell (e.g., initiated cell, Figure 1). The transformed phenotype, however, is repressed until whatever restraining influences being exerted on the cell are overcome. Many compounds, known as promoters, have been identified which can release the initiated cell from these influences resulting in a cell expressing the transformed phenotype (e.g., transformed cell, Figure 1). One mechanism by which a promoter may act is to depress the immune system which may be restraining the phenotypic expression of initiated cells. Alternatively, natural resistance mechanisms could be operative at the transformed cell stage via recognition of the transformed phenotype, and thus prevent tumor outgrowth. This process is what is thought to occur in many of the tumor dormancy models (Weinhold, Goldstein and Wheelock, 1979; Wheelock, Weinhold, Ingenito and Goldstein, 1980; Weinhold and Wheelock, 1982). We believe that agents which interfere with these proposed mechanisms may facilitate tumor outgrowth.

One prototype promoter which our laboratory has been investigating for its effects on immunological and natural resistance mechanisms is 12-o-tetradecanoyl-phorbol-13-acetate (TPA). TPA is a potent promoter isolated from croton oil which has been demonstrated to potentiate the action of carcinogens in the mouse skin model (for reviews see Van Duuren, 1969; Blumberg, 1980; Blumberg, 1981). TPA has also been shown to enhance transformation in vitro following exposure of fibroblasts to polycyclic aromatic hydrocarbons or to oncogenic viruses (Lasne, Gentil and Chouroulinkov, 1974; Fisher, Weinstein, Eisenberg and Ginsberg, 1978). The immunological effects associated with in vitro exposure to TPA include ability to induce lymphocyte mitogenesis (Touraine, Hadden, Touraine, Hadden, Estensen and Good, 1977), to stimulate cap formation in response to Con A (Kwong and Mueller, 1982), to inhibit the stimulation of cytotoxic T-cells (Devens and Hannon, 1982), to inhibit (Keller, 1979; Fish, Baxter and Bash, 1981; Fredrickson and Bennett, 1982) or to enhance (Laskin, Laskin, Kessler, Weinstein and Carchman, 1981; Grimm, Barlin, Leser, Kramer and Gemsa, 1980) cytotoxic effector mechanisms and induce macrophage phagocytosis (Laskin, Laskin, Weinstein and Carchman, 1980). These numerous effects of TPA in vitro on the immune system have prompted us to investigate what effects TPA may have on immune function and resistance mechanisms in an in vivo model.

RESULTS

Adult B6C3F1 female mice were given biweekly subcutaneous injections of TPA for two weeks at an exposure level of 0.05, 0.5, 5 and 10μg/g body weight resulting in a total exposure of .02, 2, 20 or 40μg/g. The immune function and resistance assays were performed 3-5 days following the last exposure as described in detail (Luster, Dean and Moore, 1982a).

One general indicator of immunosuppression which was examined involved changes in the percent T and B cells present in the spleens of TPA treated mice. As can be seen in Table 1, TPA treatment resulted in a depression of both T and B cells in the spleen as measured by the appearance of T-cell (Thy-1) and B-cell (IgG) markers on the cell surface.

Table 1 Effect of TPA on lymphocyte surface markers and lymphoproliferative responses.

Dose of TPA ($\mu g/g$)	% of Cells Staining +		CPM of ^{3}H-TdR Incorporation X 10^{-3} §				
	Antimouse Thymocyte	Anti-IgG	Media	PHA	Con A	LPS	MLC
0	50.3	44.0	0.5	41.5	66.3	10.7	14.0
2	ND	ND	0.8[a] (+60)	47.4 (+14)	69.0 (+4)	11.3 (+5)	15.4 (+10)
20	ND	ND	1.7[a] (+240)	36.3 (-13)	53.1 (-20)	9.3 (-13)	15.0 (+7)
40	20.5[b] (-59)	36.0[a] (-18)	2.5[b] (+400)	26.6[a] (-36)	32.5[a] (-51)	5.9[a] (-45)	9.6[a] (-31)

[a]Significantly different from controls at $p < 0.05$.

[b]Significantly different from controls at $p < 0.01$.

ND = Not done. §Percent change relative to control indicated in parentheses.

While the numbers of T and B cells can give some indication as to the immunocompetance of an organism, it is also necessary to examine the functional integrity of the cells which are present. For example, it has been shown that following cyclophosphamide treatment the spleen cells which remain are impaired in their ability to respond to mitogenic stimulation (Dean, Padarathsingh and Jerrels, 1979). Thus, we examined the ability of T and/or B cells to proliferate in response to mitogens and the ability of leukocytes to proliferate in response to alloantigens in one-way mixed leukocyte cultures (MLC). As can be seen in Table 1, spontaneous proliferation of spleen cells was enhanced in a dose dependent manner in TPA treated mice. In contrast, the lymphoproliferative response to the T-cell mitogens phytohemagglutinin (PHA) and concanavalin A (Con-A) and the MLC response were significantly depressed at the 40 $\mu g/g$ dose. The lymphoproliferative response of B-cells to _E. coli_ lipopolysaccharide (LPS) was also decreased at the highest dose.

While the lymphoproliferation data were indicative of a generalized suppression of the immune system, it was still necessary to ascertain the ability of the immune cells to function in a normal manner _in vivo_. This was accomplished by examining the ability of the mice to mount a humoral response to the T-dependent antigen sheep red blood cells (SRBC) and the T-independent antigen LPS. As can be seen in Table 2, TPA severely depressed (up to 65%) the ability of the mice to respond to the T-dependent antigen, SRBC, while having little effect on the LPS response (only a 35% decrease). This would indicate that the TPA appeared to have a more profound effect on T-cells, probably T-helper cells, than it does on B-cells. This may occur by a direct effect on T-cells or at the level of cell-cell cooperation between T and B cells.

Table 2 Effect of TPA on antibody responses and macrophage function.

Dose of TPA (μg/g)	PFC/10^6 Spleen Cells ± SEM §		% Change of Phagocytosis of SRBC by Macrophages	% Cytostasis of MBL-2 by Macrophages
	SRBC	LPS		
0	1.61 ± 0.14	2.62 ± 0.36	0	0
2	0.57 ± 0.03[a] (-65%)	ND	+4	-6
20	0.58 ± 0.07[a] (-64%)	1.80 ± 0.24 (-32%)	-8	+82[a]
40	0.75 ± 0.13[a] (-54%)	1.78 ± 0.10 (-32%)	-48[b]	+89[a]

[a] Significantly different from control at $p < 0.01$.

[b] Significantly different from control at $p < 0.05$.

ND = Not done. §Percent change relative to control indicated in parentheses.

Table 2 also summarizes the results of two assays of macrophage function, phagocytosis and cytostasis. *In vivo* exposure to TPA affects the ability of macrophages to phagocytize SRBC *in vitro*, which is contrary to *in vitro* exposure in which phagocytosis is enhanced (Laskin *et al*, 1980). *In vivo* exposure to TPA also activates macrophages for cytostasis of tumor cells *in vitro*. This activation is a characteristic associated with inflammatory macrophages (Adams and Dean, 1982). The *in vivo* relevance of this cytostatic effect has yet to be determined, since it does not appear to influence resistance to tumor challenge (see below).

The last group of experiments to assess the integrity of the immune system in TPA treated mice involved tumor susceptibility assays (Table 3). Mice challenged with an LD20 of the sarcoma PYB6 subsequent to exposure to 20 or 40 μg/g of TPA had an increased frequency with a shorter latency period (data not shown) than controls. In addition, mice challenged i.v. with the B16F10 malanoma cells, a tumor which preferentially localizes in the lungs, exhibited an increased number of tumor colonies in the lungs at all doses of TPA tested in comparison to controls. Also included in Table 3 are the results of in vitro natural cytotoxicity studies against the tumor target YAC-1, which is the standard method for measuring natural killer cell activity (Ortaldo, Bonnard and Herberman, 1977). It is evident from the results that a marked reduction in the spontaneous cytotoxicity of splenic lymphocytes to tumor target cells existed at all the doses of TPA examined, which is consistent with the results of the B16F10 challenge data. To further assess the in vivo role of the depressed NK response, mice were intraveneously challenged with 5-iodo-2'-deoxyuridine-labelled B16F10 melanoma cells, and the

Table 3 Effect of TPA on tumor susceptibility and NK activity.

Dose of TPA (μg/g)	PYB6 Challenge (% Tumor)	B16F10 Challenge (No. Nodules/ Lung ± SEM)	NK Assay (% Cytolysis)	In Vivo Clearance of ^{125}IUdR Labeled B16F10 Cells/Lung		
				CPM x 10^{-3} ± SEM 0.5 hrs	3 hrs	% Change
0	23	15 ±1.2	20.3	50.9 ±10.0	18.1 ±1.9	-64.5[b]
0.2	ND	ND	ND	66.6 ±4.6	41.6 ±16.0	-37.5
2	37	41 ± 5[a]	2.7[b]	ND	ND	ND
20	57[b]	68 ± 4[a]	3.3[b]	63.1 ±8.9	46.9 ±9.3	-25.7
40	61[b]	81 ± 7[a]	4.4[b]	ND	ND	ND

[a] Significantly different from controls at $p < 0.05$.

[b] Significantly different from controls at $p < 0.01$.

ND = Not done.

amount of label present in the lungs at 0.5 and 3 hours was measured (Table 3). The results demonstrate that although initial deposition was the same in both control and TPA exposed mice, the normal mice had removed 83% of the tumor cells by 3 hours, while no significant clearance of tumor cells occurred in TPA treated mice. The initial in vivo lysis of B16F10 cells is thought to be mediated by NK cells (Hanna and Fidler, 1980).

DISCUSSION

While the mechanism by which TPA exerts its immunological effects is currently unknown, it would appear from the present study that T-lymphocyte dependent functions are the most susceptible to the effects of TPA. T-cell suppression was evidenced by the antibody plaque cell data where the T-dependent response was significantly depressed by TPA exposure while the assay for B-cell function (i.e., the LPS response) was not affected. It remains to be determined at what level the T-cell response has been suppressed; i.e. has there been an induction of T-suppressor cells, has the TPA directly acted on the T-helper cell population, or are accessory cell functions impaired? One possible explanation for the selectivity of TPA for lymphoid cells is suggested by the recent observation of Estensen, DeHoogh and Cole (1980) that peripheral blood lymphocytes have a binding protein for this molecule.

It has been previously demonstrated that the ability of many tumors to metastasize, including B16, is directly affected by alterations in NK cell activity (Reid, Minato, Gresser, Holland, Kadish and Bloom, 1981; Talmadge et al, 1980a; Talmadge et al, 1980b). The results of this study reaffirms these findings since both NK activity and B16 lung tumor foci were significantly altered at the lowest dose of TPA tested. As these assays are probably more indicative of tumor resistance than the other assays examined, these results would lend support to the hypothesis that one mechanism by which promoters may be operating is via suppression of natural resistance mechanisms. In addition, it should be emphasized that the immunosuppressive effects caused by TPA occur at dosage levels which do not cause clinical signs of toxicity but are tumor promoting.

One question which remains to be answered involves the reversibility of the immunotoxic effects of TPA on the immune system. As was previously stated, one characteristic of promoters is the transient and reversible nature of their effects. It has been demonstrated that following ablation of the immune system by sub-lethal irradiation, normal T and B cell functions are regenerated (Anderson and Warner, 1976). It would be interesting to determine if the effects noted in the current study are also reversible, with particular reference to the natural resistance assays. If this was found to be the case it would lend more support to the idea that some promoters may act by compromising immunocompetence.

The results demonstrated with TPA may not be unique to this promoting agent. Other chemicals of environmental concern with known promotional ability (such as urethane and TCDD) have recently been demonstrated to cause immunosuppression in the natural resistance assays utilized in the current study (Luster, Dean and Boorman, 1982b). This should not be construed to mean that promoters exert their effect solely by suppression of the immune system. Indeed, immunosuppression may be only one facet of the effects of certain promoters. However, it is interesting to note that the immunoassays which most closely analyze natural resistance mechanisms, i.e., B16 challenge and the NK assay, are also those which are the most sensitive to the effects of TPA. Much more work remains to be done before any firm conclusions can be reached on the interrelationship of tumor promoters to immunosurveillance in the mechanisms of chemical carcinogenesis.

In summary, the current study with the tumor promoter TPA demonstrates that: 1) in vivo exposure to TPA suppresses the ability of T and B cells to proliferate in response to appropriate mitogenic stimuli; 2) the cell-cell cooperation between T and B cells as measured by the mouse's ability to mount an antibody response to the T-dependent antigen SRBC was depressed; 3) the susceptibility of TPA-treated mice to tumor challenge is compromised; and 4) the natural resistance of mice as measured by NK activity is severely depressed by TPA exposure.

REFERENCES

ADAMS, D.O. and DEAN, J.H. (1982) In: Natural Mechanisms of Immunity II. (ed. Herberman, R.) Academic Press, New York.

ANDERSON, R.E. and WARNER, N.L. (1976) Ionizing radiation and the immune response. Adv. Immunol. 24, 215.

BALDWIN, R.W. (1973) Immunological aspects of chemical carcinogenesis. Adv. Can. Res. 18, 1.

BERNBLUM, I. (1975) In: Cancer Vol 1 (ed. Becher, F.F.) Plenum Press, New York, p. 323.

BLUMBERG, P.M. (1980) In vitro studies on the mode of action of the phorbol esters, potent tumor promoters: Part I. CRC Crit. Rev. Toxicol. 8, 153.

BLUMBERG, P.M. (1981) In vitro studies on the mode of action of the phorbol esters, potent tumor promoters: Part II. CRC Crit. Rev. Toxicol. 9, 199.

BURNET, F.M. (1970) The concept of immunological surveillance. Prog. Exp. Tumor Res. 13, 1.

DEAN, J.H., McCOY, J.L., LEWIS, D., APPELLA, E. and LAW, L.W. (1975) Studies of lymphocyte stimulation by intact tumor cell and solubilized tumor antigen. Int. J. Cancer 16, 465.

DEAN, J.H., PADARATHSINGH, M.L. and JERRELS, T.R. (1979) Application of immunocompetence assays for defining immunosuppression. Ann. N.Y. Acad. Sci. 320, 579.

DEVENS, B.H. and HANNON, M.A. (1982) Differential effects of tumor promoters on immune cell subpopulations. Fed. Proc. 41, 331.

ESTENSEN, R.D., DeHOOGH, D.K. and COLE, C.F. (1980) Binding of [^{3}H] 12-O-tetradecanoylphorbol-13-acetate to intact human peripheral blood lymphocytes. Cancer Res. 40, 1119.

FISH, L.A., BAXTER, C.S. and BASH, J.A. (1981) Inhibition of macrophage-induced tumor cell cytostasis and cytolysis by tumor-promoting phorbol diesters. Toxicology 19, 127.

FISHER, P.B., WEINSTEIN, B., EISENBERG, D. and GINSBERG, H.S. (1978) Interactions between adenovirus, a tumor promoter, and chemical carcinogens in transformation of rat embryo cell cultures. Proc. Nat. Acad. Sci. 75, 2311.

FREDRICKSON, G.G. and BENNETT, M. (1982) Suppression of the cytotoxic response of mouse lymphocytes to syngeneic tumor cells by tumor-promoting phorbol esters. Cancer Res. 42, 3601.

GREENBERG, A.H. and GREENE, M. (1976) Non-adaptive rejection of small tumour inocula as a model of immune surveillance. Nature 264, 356.

GRIMM, W., BARLIN, E., LESER, H.G., KRAMER, W. and GEMSA, D. (1980) Induction of tumor cytostatic macrophages by 12-O-tetradecanoylphorbol-13-acetate (TPA). Clin. Immunol. and Immunopathol. 17, 617.

HANNA, N. and FIDLER, I.J. (1980) Role of natural killer cells in the destruction of circulating tumor emboli. J. Natl. Cancer Inst. 65, 801.

HERBERMAN, R.B., DJEU, J.Y., KAY, H.D., ORTALDO, J.R., RICCARDI, C., BONNARD, G.D., HOLDEN, H.T., FAGNANI, R., SANTONI, A. and PUCCETTI, P. (1979) Natural killer cells: Characteristics and regulation of activity. Immunol. Rev. 44, 43.

HERBERMAN, R.B. and ORTALDO, J.R. (1981) Natural killer cells: Their role in defenses against disease. Science 214, 24.

KAWASE, I., URDAL, D.C., BROOKS, C.G. and HENNEY, C.S. (1982) Selective depletion of NK cell activity in vivo and its effect on the growth of NK-sensitive and NK-resistant tumor cell variants. Int. J. Cancer 29, 567.

KARRE, K., KLEIN, G.O., KIESSLING, R., KLEIN, E. and RODER, J.C. (1980) In vitro NK-activity and in vivo resistance to leukemia: studies of beige, beige/nude and wild-type hosts on C57BL background. Int. J. Cancer 26, 789.

KELLER, R. (1979) Suppression of naturalantitumour defence mechanisms by phorbol esters. Nature 282, 729.

KIESSLING, R. and WIGZELL, H. (1979) Analyses of the murine NK cell as to structure, function and biological relevance. Immunol. Rev. 44, 165.

KLEIN, G. (1966) Tumor antigens. Ann. Rev. Microbiol. 20, 223.

KLEIN, G. and KLEIN, E. (1977a) Immune surveillance against virus-induced tumors and nonrejectability of spontaneous tumors: Contrasting consequences of host versus tumor evolution. Proc. Nat. Acad. Sci. 74, 2121.

KLEIN, G. and KLEIN, E. (1977b) Rejectability of virus-induced tumors and nonrejectability of spontaneous tumors: A lesson in contrasts. Transplant. Proc. 9, 1095.

KLEIN, G., SJOGREN, H.O., KLEIN, E. and HELLSTROM, K.E. (1960) Demonstration of resistance against methylcholanthrene-induced sarcomas in the primary autochthonous host. Cancer Res. 20, 1561.

KRIPKE, M.L. and BORSOS, T. (1974) Immunosuppression and carcinogenesis. Isr. J. Med. Sci. 10, 888.

KWONG, C.H. and MUELLER, G.C. (1982) Antagonism of concanavalin A capping in phorbol ester activated lymphocytes by calmodulin inhibitors and certain amino acid esters. Cancer Res. 42, 2115.

LASKIN, D.L., LASKIN, J.D., WEINSTEIN, I.B. and CARCHMAN, R.A. (1980) Modulation of phagocytosis by tumor promoters and epidermal growth factor in normal and transformed macrophages. Cancer Res. 40, 1028.

LASKIN, D.L., LASKIN, J.D., KESSLER, F.K., WEINSTEIN, I.B. and CARCHMAN, R.A. (1981) Enhancement of macrophage-induced cytotoxicity by phorbol ester tumor promoters. Cancer Res. 41, 4523.

LASNE, C., GENTIL, A. and CHOUROULINKOV, I. (1974) Two-stage malignant transformation of rat fibroblasts in tissue culture. Nature 247, 490.

LUSTER, M.I., DEAN, J.H. and MOORE, J.A. (1982a) In: Principles and Methods in Toxicology (ed. Hayes, A.W.) Raven Press, New York, p. 561.

LUSTER, M.I., DEAN, J.H. and BOORMAN, G. (1982b) Immune functions in methyl and ethyl carbamate treated mice. Clin. Exptl. Immunol. 50, 223.

MASTRANGELO, M.J., LAUCIUS, J.F. and OUTZEN, H.C. (1974) Fundamental concepts in tumor immunology: A brief review. Semin. Oncol. 1, 291.

OLD, L.J., BOYSE, E.A., CLARKE, D.A. and CRESSWELL, E.A. (1962) Antigenic properties of chemically induced tumors. Ann. N.Y. Acad. Sci. 101, 80.

ORTALDO, J.R., BONNARD, G.D. and HERBERMAN, R.B. (1977) Cytotoxic reactivity of human lymphocyte cultured in vitro. J. Immunol. 119, 1351.

OUTZEN, H.C. (1980) Development of carcinogen-induced skin tumors in mice with varied states of immune capacity. Int. J. Cancer, 26, 87.

OUTZEN, H.C. and CUSTER, R.P. (1975) Growth of human normal and neoplastic mammary tissues in the cleared mammary fat pad of the nude mice. J. Natl. Cancer Inst. 55, 1461.

PENN, I. (1982) In: Current Problems in Cancer Vol. 6 (eds. Hickey, R.C. and Clark, R.L.) Year Book Medical Publishers, Inc., New York, p. 1.

PREHN, R.T. (1963) Tumor specific immunity to nonviral tumors. Can. Cancer Conf. 5, 387.

PREHN, R.T. and MAIN, J.M. (1957) Immunity to methylcholanthrene-induced sarcomas. J. Natl. Cancer Inst. 18, 769.

REID, L., MINATO, N., GRESSER, I., HOLLAND, J., KADISH, A. and BLOOM, B. (1981) Influence of anti-mouse interferon serum on the growth and metastasis of tumor cells persistently infected with virus and of human prostatic tumors in athymic nude mice. Proc. Nat. Acad. Sci. 78, 1171.

RODER, J.C. and DUWE, A.K. (1979) The beige mutation in the mouse selectively impairs natural killer cell function. Nature 278, 451.

SHEIL, A.G.R., MAHONY, J.F., HORVATH, J.S., JOHNSON, J.R., TILLER, D.J., STEWART, J.H. and MAY, J. (1981) Cancer following successful cadaveric donor renal transplantation. Transplant. Proc. 13, 733.

SJOGREN, H.O. (1965) Transplantation methods as a tool for detection of tumor-specific antigens. Progr. Exptl. Tumor Res. 6, 289.

STJERNSWARD. J. (1966) Host barrier and effect of carcinogen-induced immunodepression on rejection of isografted methylcholanthrene-induced sarcoma cells. J. Nat. Cancer Inst. 37, 505.

STUTMAN, O. (1978) In: The Nude Mouse in Experimental and Clinical Research (eds. Fogh, J. and Giovanella, B.) Academic Press, New York, p. 411.

TALMADGE, J.E., MEYERS, K.M., PRIEUR, D.J. and STARKEY, J.R. (1980a) Role of natural killer cells in tumor growth and metastasis: C57BL/6 normal and beige mice. J. Natl. Cancer Inst. 65, 929.

TALMADGE, J.E., MEYERS, K.M., PRIEUR, D.J. and STARKEY, J.R. (1980b) Role of NK cells in tumour growth and metastasis in beige mice. Nature 284, 622.

TOURAINE, J.L., HADDEN, J.W., TOURAINE, F., HADDEN, E.M., ESTENSEN, R. and GOOD, R.A. (1977) Phorbol myristate acetate: A mitogen selective for a T-lymphocyte subpopulation. J. Exp. Med. 145, 460.

VAN DUUREN, B.L. (1969) Tumor promoting agents in two-stage carcinogenesis. Progr. Exp. Tumor Res. 11, 31.

WARNER, N.C., WOODRUFF, M.F.A. and BURTON, R.C. (1977) Inhibition of the growth of lymphoid tumors in syngeneic athymic (nude) mice. Int. J. Cancer 20, 146.

WEINHOLD, K.J., GOLDSTEIN, L.T. and WHEELOCK, E.F. (1979) The tumor dormant state: Quantitation of L5178Y cells and hose immune responses during the establishment and course of dormancy in syngeneic DBA/2 mice. J. Exp. Med. 149, 732.

WEINHOLD, K.J. and WHEELOCK, E.F. (1982) Cross-reacting antigens on L5178Y cells which serve as targets for cytotoxic T-lymphocyte lysis during establishment of the tumor dormant state. Cancer Res. 42, 3607.

WHEELOCK, E.F., WEINHOLD, K.J., INGENITO, G.G. and GOLDSTEIN, L.T. (1980) In vivo lysis of L5178Y cells in the establishment of the tumor-dormant state in DBA/2 mice. J. Immunol. 124, 1642.

DRUG ALLERGIES:
FACTORS INFLUENCING INDUCTION AND DIAGNOSIS

Harry E. Amos
Imperial Chemical Industries Inc.
Alderly Park, Cheshire
SK10 4TJ, U.K.

It is important that the concepts embodied in the term immunotoxicity include both toxic damage to the immunological system and tissue damage brought about by activating the system. The latter is frequently referred to as hypersensitivity but its essential feature is that an untoward clinical response results from an allergic reaction i.e., antigen interacting with specific antibody or with specifically allergised cells. It must be borne in mind that an allergic reaction is an adaptive response and is biologically normal. If antigens did not activate the immunological system to make antibodies and the two interact together, the body would lack a basic defence mechanism and be unable to survive (cf severe combined immunodeficiency states).

Hypersensitivity responses resulting from allergic reactions do pose a considerable clinical hazard and are particularly worrying when xenobiotics are deliberately administered as this implies that some form of safety assessment has previously taken place. For various reasons which will be discussed, the evaluation of a compound in terms of its potential hypersensitivity risk to man is not possible at present but the science of toxicology is advancing and it is the job of an immunotoxicologist to marry these advances with those in immunology to increase confidence in safety evaluation.

INCIDENCE

Epidemiological analyses of adverse drug reaction notifications show that as many as 5% of all hospital admissions are due to drug induced disease (Nat. Acad. Sci. USA Statistics, 1971). The incidence of adverse drug effects not requiring hospital admission is likely to be very much higher, but of these it is possible only to guess the proportion which are due to hypersensitivity. Many reactions are not investigated; hypersensitivity has mechanistic implications but it is frequently used as a definitive diagnosis without corrobarative data! Thus, without a real idea of the scale of the problem which hypersensitivity to xenobiotics causes, it is difficult to promote interest in funding research of a more fundemental nature.

NATO ASI Series, Vol. G2
Immunotoxicology. Edited by P. W. Mullen

SPECIES SPECIFIC FACTORS ACCOUNTING FOR INTERSPECIES VARIATION IN DRUG RESPONSES

The use of animal models for dissecting the immunological system in man has proved to be rewarding, but attempting to equate immunogenicity data across species barriers must be done with extreme caution. Different species may process a drug to generate products which are species specific. Moreover, some products, by virtue of their chemical reactivity may be suitable antigens and induce immunological reactions which would not be induced in other species.

The now classical work of Williams and Parke (1964), in which aromatic hydroxylation was compared in several species clearly demonstrated qualitative differences as shown in Table 1. As well as differences in the amount of a particular metabolite produced there are differences in the preferred route of metabolism.

For example, imipramine is selectively degraded in man to form a nor-derivative.

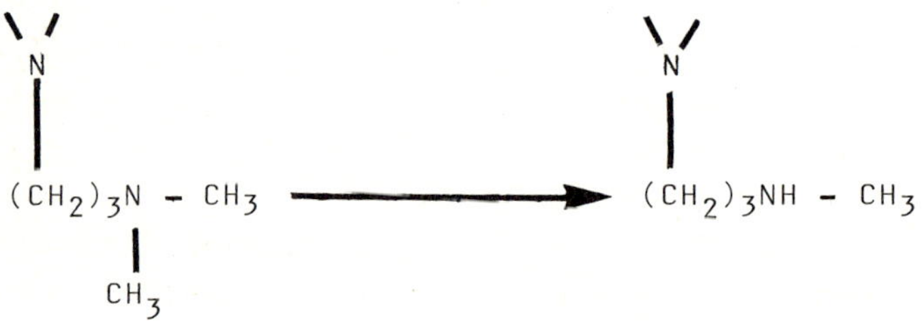

For rabbits and rats this does not occur, the preferred route of metabolism in these species is ring hydroxylation.

These examples illustrate the point that metabolic pathways along which drugs can be directed should be taken into account when an animal is chosen to model a potential event in man. Although these examples do not specifically relate to hypersensitivity, it is possible to speculate that a quantitative difference in the generation of a metabolite which could function as a hapten could influence a study designed to establish immunogenic potential.

The governing factor for interspecies variation in metabolism is the individual's genetic constitution. This is succinctly illustrated by the work of Evans, Mahgoub, Sloan, Idle and Smith (1980). They showed that even within a species (man) there is variation in the degree of debrisoquine alicyclic hydroxylation. By carrying out population studies they identified a group which were deficient in the hydroxylating enzyme and established that the trait was inherited as a single autosomal recessive.

The evidence implicating genetic constraints on metabolic processes is overwhelming, but the essential argument is whether such variation is of clinical importance. In the case of debrisoquine, failure to detoxify the parent drug into therapeutically inactive hydroxylated metabolites would clearly increase the serum half-life of the active compound, leading to predictable side effects. It has also been known for some years, that fast and slow acetylation of hydralazine exists, and that there is an association between slow acetylators and the propensity to develop drug dependent lupus erythematosus (Perry, Tan, Carmody and Sakamoto, 1970).

Evidence of genetic involvement is more difficult to find if antigenicity is the criterion, the oculomucocutaneous syndrome of practolol is probably the best example of a species specific reaction which forms metabolites capable of stimulating antibodies, but here more work would be needed to determine the determinent specificity of the response and the role played by genetics.

In addition to genetic constraints influencing the metabolism of compounds, they are also important in determining the immunological response.

GENETIC CONSTRAINT ON THE IMMUNE RESPONSE

Allowing for variation in metabolite production and the assumption that a drug or metabolite covalently bound to a protein can form an immunogenic unit, there is no guarantee that an individual will respond immunologically.

The immune response is known to be governed by a set of genes (Ir), which determine whether a particular structure can behave as an antigen (McDevitt and Chinitz, 1969). Possession of appropriate Ir genes however does not always lead to a detectable immune response, other genetic factors operate to determine the magnitude. Selective breeding experiments between mice injected with benzyl penicilloyl-polylysine showed that two distinct permutations emerged; high and low responses (Levine and Vaz, 1970). It has been suggested that the genetic control which characterizes the level of reactivity is connected with antigen processing by macrophages (Biozzi, Stiffel, Mouton, Bouthillier and Decreusfond, 1972).

The discussion so far has been concerned with factors which govern variation between and within species of antigen formation and the effective response. It must be stressed again that this is a biologically normal event. Provided a drug forms an immunogenic unit, it is likely that antibody production will occur in most individuals, but clearly not all develop hypersensitivity reactions. Thus, there must be an "at risk" group if it could only be identified. One attempt at identifying individuals potentially capable of developing hypersensitivity reactions to drugs has been to study HLA phenotypes. Spengler and de Weck (1977) phenotyped forty-six patients with demonstrable clinical and serological evidence of penicillin allergy and were able to show only that antigens Bw35, B18 and A28 appeared to be more common in the allergic patients than in controls, but without any statistical significance. There is no further evidence linking HLA phenotypes with a susceptibility to develop hypersensitivity response to drugs, but clearly further information would be of great value.

EVIDENCE OF IMMUNOLOGICAL RESPONSES SPECIFIC FOR DRUG METABOLITES

Drugs are metabolised by a heterogenous group of enzymes collectively termed mixed-function oxidases. They are located within the microsomal fraction of the endoplasmic reticulum and are concentrated mainly in the liver, but most tissues have a degree of metabolising capacity and it is conceivable that local metabolism may be a significant factor in specific organ toxicity. It is also possible to speculate that localisation of a metabolite with antigenic properties at the site of metabolic conversion may account for the tissue fixation of specific antibiotics.

General evidence that metabolic products from first phase metabolism can induce specific antibodies is limited to three examples; β-lactam antibiotics, practolol and halothane.

β-Lactam Antibodies

Drugs derived from the 6-amino derivative of penicillanic acid or the acyl derivative of 7-amino cephalosporonic acid readily undergo a number of chemical and enzymic modifications to yield products which have specificity for circulating antibodies.

The penicilloyl determinant forming an amide linkage between the carbonyl function of the β-lactam ring and nucleophilic side chains of proteins is the major configuration for stimulating an antibody response to penicillin.

Antibodies have also been characterized for other biotransformed products. For example, reactive sulphydryls formed from the thioether can generate mixed disulphides with proteins containing the penicilloyl determinant. Further conversion to the penamaldyl and penicillamyl determinant is also possible. Antibodies to each of these determinants have been reported.

Although the antigenicity of cephalosporins has not been as extensively studied as that of penicillin, basic similarities between the structure and chemical behaviour make it likely that cephalosporin(s) and penicillin(s) are comparable in their antigenic properties. There is no doubt that minor determinants of penicillin can stimulate IgE antibodies and are responsible for a proportion of reported anaphylactic reactions.

Halothane

Halothane is a fluorinated hydrocarbon used as a volatile anaesthetic and there is a clinical association between repeated use of the drug and hepatic damage. Minor asymptomatic deviations of serum transaminases have been reported to occur in about 20% of patients receiving repeated exposure (Trowell, Peto and Crampton-Smith, 1975) and in about 1 in 35,000 patients a severe hepatic necrosis develops (Strunin, 1977).

The possibility that a hypersensitivity mechanism may be involved in the pathogenesis arose following a number of epidemiological observations.

(a) Accelerated onset after more than one halothane exposure (Inman and Mushin, 1974).
(b) Unexplained post-operative pyrexia following exposure (Trey, Lipworth and Chalmers, 1968).
(c) Frequent past history of allergy.

Investigations have added some support to the clinical observations in that antibodies to normal liver membrane components have been found in the sera of affected patients (Jensen, 1979). Attempts to obtain more definitive evidence by demonstrating halothane specific antibodies have been unrewarding.

The first observation that a minor metabolite may be involved in the production of hepatic necrosis was the finding that a product of halothane metabolism via an oxidative pathway was capable of rendering rabbit hepatocytes antigenic (Neuburger, Mieli-Vergani, Tredger, Davis and Williams, 1980). Antibodies to the altered hepatocytes have been characterized and appear to be restricted to patients with halothane induced liver necrosis (Vergani, Mieli-Vergani and Alberti, 1980).

The metabolite has not yet been fully identified nor have antibodies with metabolite specificity, but a body of evidence is growing which supports a hypothesis postulating that necrosis results from direct interaction of an antibody with halothane altered hepatocyte membranes. The possibility that an antibody mediated cytotoxic reaction may also be involved stemmed from finding that the "antibody" was able to induce normal lymphocytes to become cytotoxic to halothane treated hepatocytes (Vergani *et al*, 1980).

Practolol

The cardioselective β-receptor blocking agent, practolol, induced in a small number of patients a syndrome defined as "oculomucocutaneous". As the name implies the main sites of tissue damage were confined to the eyes and serosal surfaces including the peritoneum and skin.

Epidemiological studies identified two factors which suggested that the tissue damage might not be due to a direct toxic effect of the drug but might implicate an immunological element in the pathogenesis. These were: (a) the syndrome was not dose related and (b) incidence was low. Support for an immunological role came from a demonstration of tissue specific auto-antibodies in sera of patients with the syndrome (Amos, Brigden and McKerron, 1975).

Despite numerous attempts to identify a practolol specific antibody, however, none were successful. A possibility that a metabolite might be antigenic was investigated by Amos, Lake and Atkinson (1977). The reasoning was based on circumstantial evidence outlined above and the fact that no animal model could be found for the adverse response, indicating that the oculomucocutaneous syndrome was species specific for man. Using an *in vitro* mixed-function oxygenase generating system to metabolise practolol, Amos *et al* (1977) were able to demonstrate an antibody which reacted with products of the metabolism. Subsequent experiments showed that metabolite specific antibodies could be demonstrated not only in patients with the syndrome, but also in patients taking practolol with no overt clinical signs of the defined tissue damage (Amos, Lake and Artis, 1978). Whether or not these latter patients would eventually develop the syndrome as a result of antigen-antibody interaction will have to remain an open question.

PSEUDO-ALLERGIC REACTIONS

The term "pseudo-allergic" refers to reactions which mimic signs and symptoms of allergic disorders but without involvement of immunological mechanisms. Thus the inducing compound does not act as an antigen. This complicates diagnosis because the final pathway, for both hypersensitivity reactions and pseudo-allergic responses, may be the same. Distinction can be made only after carrying out an investigative programme.

The main thrust of experimental work into pseudo-allergic reactions has been with compounds which induce signs of clinical anaphylaxis, such as synacthen (Jacques and Bruggen, 1969) and intravenous anaesthetic drugs (Lorenz, Doenicke, Halbach, Krumey and Werle, 1969). An important target for these compounds is the complement system, and it is thought that activation of mast cells by complement components liberated during the fixation sequence is the mechanism of the anaphylactoid reaction.

INVESTIGATING SUSPECTED DRUG ALLERGIES

A pragmatic clinical approach to a suspected drug allergy would be to stop the drug and substitute an alternative preparation; there is nearly always one available, but it can be dangerous in blindly adopting such a policy. Care must be exercised to ensure that there is not likely to be any immunological cross reactivity with the substituted drug. This of course implies that the allergy has to be correctly diagnosed in the first place — a procedure that might require some type of investigation.

Amos (1980) suggested that a comprehensive approach to investigating suspected drug allergies should consist of a four phase study.

Phase I

This consists of a detailed clinical appraisal which includes a specific drug history and an assessment of any epidemiological data which may be available on a particular drug.

Phase 2

The essence of a phase 2 approach is to identify any factor which might herald an immunological response. Demonstration of auto-antibodies, changes in immunoglobulin or complement levels could show that a drug is capable of pertubating the immunological system with subsequent involvement in the pathogenesis of the observed adverse effect.

Phase 3

This is the most important phase of the scheme and often the most difficult. It is aimed at obtaining evidence of antibodies or actively allergised cells which have specificity for the drug or drug products. Two approaches to phase 3 are possible, *in vivo* skin or provocation tests and *in vitro* procedures. The choice of investigative manoeuvres will depend on the circumstances of each individual case, but clearly a combination of skin tests and laboratory studies is preferable.

The difficulty encountered in trying to show a drug specific immunological response is in deciding which form of drug determinant is to be expressed in the system. Coupling the drug to some immunological indicator particle is usually a necessary step in any *in vitro* test, and if the result is positive, it should be possible to prove antibody specificity. If a negative result is produced interpretation is more difficult and it may be necessary to explore alternative determinant configurations before concluding that no drug antibodies are present.

Phase 4

The last phase of the investigation is to provide data on the relevance of a specific immunological response to the induced clinical effect. As mentioned in an earlier section, drugs are small molecular weight compounds and will, if the conditions are favourable, stimulate antibody production. The demonstration of antibodies, therefore, is not sufficient in itself to justify a diagnosis of drug allergy. There is no good procedure for obtaining relevant data, but a well conducted provocation study, coupled to a measurement of antibody titres, is sometimes useful. The aim would be to link a rise in antibody titres to exacerbation of the clinical signs.

CONCLUSION

The difficulties outlined in this paper may at first sight seem insurmountable. The diversity of factors influencing an individual's ability to respond adversely to a drug could deter the most diligent of investigators, and used, with some justification, as an excuse for doing nothing. Research however, in related fields, particularly genetics and drug metabolism, is expanding very rapidly and the immunotoxicologist must be ready to respond to any advance which could lead to a re-evaluation of safety assessment.

REFERENCES

AMOS, H.E. (1980) In: Recent Advances in Clinical Immunology, (ed. R.A. Thompson) Churchill Livingstone, Edinburgh, p. 221.

AMOS, H.E., BRIGDEN, W.D. and McKERRON, R.A. (1975) Untoward effects associated with practolol: Demonstration of antibody binding to epithelial tissue. Br. Med. J. 1, 598.

AMOS, H.E., LAKE, B.G. and ATKINSON, H.A.C. (1977) Allergic drug reactions: An *in vitro* model using a mixed function oxidase complex to demonstrate antibodies with specificity for a practolol metabolite. Clinical Allergy 7, 423.

AMOS, H.E., LAKE, B.G. and ARTIS, J. (1978) Possible role of antibody specific for a practolol metabolite in the pathogenesis of oculo-musocutaneous syndrome. Br. Med. J. 1, 402.

BIOZZI, G., STIFFEL, C., MOUTON, D., BOUTHILLIER, Y. and DECREUSEFOND, C. (1972) Cytodynamics of the immune response in two lines of mice genetically selected for "high" and "low" antibody synthesis. J. Exp. Med. 135, 1071.

EVANS, D.A.P., MAHGOUB, A., SLOAN, T.P., IDLE, J.R. and SMITH, R.L. (1980) A family and population study of the genetic polymorphism of debrisoquine oxidation in a white British population. J. Med. Genet. 17, 102.

INMAN, W.H.W. and MUSHIN, W.W. (1974) Jaundice after repeated exposure to halothane: An analysis of reports to the committee on safety of medicines. Br. Med. J. 1, 5.

JAQUES, R. and BRUGGER, M. (1969) Synthetic polypeptides related to corticotrophin acting as histamine liberators. Pharmacology 2, 361.

JENSEN, D. (1979) In: Immune Reactions in Liver Disease (eds. Eddleston, A.L.W.F.. Weber, J.C.P., Williams, R.) Pitman Medical, Tunbridge Wells, p.265.

LEVINE, B.B. and VAZ, N.M. (1970) Effect of combinations of inbred strain, antigen, and antigen dose on immune responsiveness and reagin production in the mouse. Int. Arch. Allergy. Appl. Immunol. 39, 156.

LORENZ, W., DOENICKE, A., HALBACH, S., KRUMEY, I. and WERLE, E. (1969) Histaminfreisetzung and magensaftsekretion bei narkosen mit propanidid (Epontol). Klin. Wschr. 47, 154.

McDEVITT, M.O. and CHINITZ, H. (1969) Genetic control of the antibody response relationship between immune response and histocompatibility (H-2) type. Science 163, 1207.

NEUBERGER, J.M., MIELI-VERGANI, G., TREDGER, M., DAVIS, M. and WILLIAMS, R. (1980) Oxidative metabolism of halothane in the immuno-pathogenesis of the associated liver damage (abstract). Gut 21, 467.

PERRY, H.M., TAN, E.M., CARMODY, S. and SAKAMOTO, A. (1970) Relationship of acetyl transferase activity to antinuclear antibodies and toxic symptoms in hypertensive patients treated with hydralazine. J. Lab. Clin. Med. 76, 114.

SPENGLER, H. and DeWECK, A.L. (1977) Evaluation of genetic control of the immune response to penicillin in man. Monogr. Allergy 11, 116.

STRUNIN, L. (1977) In: The Liver and Anaesthesia, London, W.B. Saunders Co., p. 166.

TREY, C., LIPWORTH, L., CHALMERS, T.C. (1968) Fulminant hepatic failure. New Eng. J. Med. 279, 798.

TROWELL, J., PETO, R. and CRAMPTON-SMITH (1975) Controlled trial of repeated halothane anaesthetics in patients with carcinoma of the uterine cervix treated with radium. Lancet 1, 821.

VERGANI, D., MIELI-VERGANI, G. and ALBERTI, A. (1980) Antibodies to the surface of halothane-altered rabbit hepatocytes in patients with severe halothane-associated hepatitis. New Eng. J. Med. 303, 66.

WILLIAMS, R.T. and PARKE, D.V. (1964) The metabolic fate of drugs. Ann. Rev. Pharmacol. 4, 85.

IMMUNOPHARMACOKINETICS:
THE PHARMACOKINETICS AND PHARMACODYNAMICS OF IMMUNOREGULATING DRUGS

Leslie Z. Benet, Udo F. Legler, Sue Y. Tsang
Brigitte M. Frey and Felix J. Frey

Department of Pharmacy
University of California
San Francisco, CA 94143, U.S.A.

Although immunosuppressive agents have been utilized extensively in a number of patient populations, little pharmacokinetic information has been available concerning the absorption and distribution of these compounds and even less information is available relating the efficacy and toxicity of these drugs to pharmacokinetic measurements. Studies in this area may be categorized under the heading immunopharmacokinetics, which may be defined as the study of the rate processes of absorption, distribution, metabolism and excretion of immunoregulatory (immunosuppressive and immunostimulating) drugs and their corresponding immunologic efficacious of toxic response (Benet, Frey, Ding and Frey, 1981). Studies in our laboratory, over the past few years, have concentrated on defining the immunopharmacokinetics of prednisone/prednisolone and azathioprine (AZA)/6-mercaptopurine (6MP), the most commonly used immunosuppressive agents. We developed sensitive and specific high pressure liquid chromatographic assays for these compounds (Frey, Frey and Benet, 1979; Ding and Benet, 1979) which allowed us to measure active drug and metabolites in animals (Ding and Benet, 1979; Frey, Frey, Greither and Benet, 1980) and man (Ding, Gambertoglio, Amend, Birnbaum and Benet, 1980; Frey, Amend, Lozada, Frey, Holford and Benet, 1981a; Legler, Frey and Benet, 1982). However, the kinetic description of these highly metabolized immunosuppressive drugs will not be particularly useful unless the pharmacokinetic parameters can be related to measures of the pharmacodynamic effect. Since it is quite difficult to define any quantitative measures of efficacy and toxicity for immunoregulating agents when the whole patient is considered, intermediate measures of immunologic effects have been sought.

In recent years much information has accumulated regarding the functions of a large number of cell types in the control of the immune system. The cells involved include T lymphocytes which act in cellular immune reactions; B lymphocytes and their plasma cell progeny, which

NATO ASI Series, Vol. G2
Immunotoxicology. Edited by P. W. Mullen

act through the production of immunoglobulins and which function in humoral immune reactions; macrophages, which are probably involved in a variety of effector mechanisms; polymorphonuclear leukocytes and mast cells. It is now clear that no particular cell type is responsible for overall control of these mechanisms. However, an important role is ascribed to the T cell which in addition to its own effector role in cell mediated immunity, also has important functions in controlling the activities of B cells through mechanisms which are described under the term "lymphocyte cooperation". Helper and suppressor T cell subclasses have now been described. Therefore, when describing alterations in immune mechanisms, it is clearly of importance to discuss the particular cell types which are involved.

For AZA and 6MP evidence points to a specific, or at least predominant role for these drugs in affecting T cell activity. As extensively reviewed by Bach (1975) this conclusion rests essentially on the findings that these agents appear to be more active both in man and in rodents on T cell-mediated responses (mixed lymphocyte reaction, blast formation by antigens or non-specific stimulants, cell mediated lymphotoxicity, delayed hypersensitivity and organ graft rejection) rather than on humoral antibody production. The literature on the effects of corticosteroids on lymphocyte function in animals and man is extensive (Fauci, 1979). Although it has been well established that corticosteroids can suppress lymphocyte blastogenic responses _in vitro_ (Fauci, Dale and Balow, 1976) it is still debated whether direct suppression of lymphocyte proliferation is a major mechanism of immunosuppressive action for _in vivo_ corticosteroids. More recent observations, as reviewed by Fauci (1979), however, suggest that corticosteroid-induced suppression of blastogenic responses may have important immunoregulatory implications. Ilfeld, Krakauer and Blaese (1977) have demonstrated that physiologic concentrations of corticosteroids markedly suppress the autologous mixed lymphocyte reaction between T cells and B cell-enriched suspensions without any suppression of the allogeneic mixed lymphocyte reaction (MLR). This suggests that corticosteroids may have a physiologic role in the _in vivo_ regulation of T cell autoreactivity.

To quantify the inhibition of T cell function by immunosuppressive drugs, Bach (1975) studied and described the inhibition of rosette formation using a mouse system. We believed that an _in vitro_ test of human T cell function would be a more desirable and probably more relevant tool for assessing immunosuppressive activity in human plasma. Cochrum, Salvatierra, Perkins and Belzer (1975) have previously demonstrated a good relation between intensity of the MLR and the survival of renal allografts. Thus, we pursued the inhibition of the MLR as a potential model for quantifying immunosuppressive activity in plasma, especially in renal allograft recipients.

We have recently described a simple and reproducible in vitro measure of immunosuppressive activity which varies as a function of time following doses of prednisolone and AZA to patients (Frey, Frey, Benet and Cochrum, 1980a). We wished to increase the percent plasma used in the MLC so that greater amounts of immunosuppressive drugs would be available to inhibit the MLR, a condition closer to that found in vivo, and thus provide a more responsive pharmacodynamic measurement to correlate with drug kinetics. Initial studies indicated that for prednisolone and AZA, a significantly greater area under the inhibition-time curve and a prolongation of detectable immunosuppressive activity could be obtained when 50% plasma was added to the MLCs rather than 10% plasma. In addition, there was slightly less variability in replicate measurements for the 50% plasma MLCs. We developed a quantitative measure of immunosuppression which appears to be related to pharmacokinetics. This measure, the area under the inhibition-time curve (Frey, Frey, Holford, Lozada and Benet, 1982) is calculated using the trapezoidal rule in a manner similar to that for the common pharmacokinetic parameter, area under the plasma concentration time curve. One of the major findings (Frey et al, 1980a), which allowed us to develop a reasonable measure of immunosuppression, was the fact that maximum inhibitory effects for prednisolone and AZA on tritiated thymidine incorporation occur at day three of the MLC incubation as opposed to day five, the time for maximum tritiated thymidine incorporation. The most probable explanation may be that at various time points of the MLR, different subpopulations of lymphocytes are active, with different sensitivities to plasma containing immunosuppressive compounds. This finding may also explain why previous workers were unable to obtain reproducible measures of immunosuppression using the usual procedures for the MLR.

To gain a better understanding of the kinetics of T cell subsets as well as the influence of prednisolone, we studied the induction kinetics of human suppressor cells in the MLR. We found that suppressor cells are apparently generated in the MLCs between days 1 and 4, and as expected, their genesis is not affected by usual therapeutic concentrations of prednisolone (Frey, Frey, Cochrum and Benet, 1980b).

PREDNISOLONE/PREDNISONE

The pharmacokinetics of prednisolone and prednisone were reviewed through 1979 by Pickup (1979) and Gambertoglio, Amend and Benet (1980).

These reviewers concluded that the available studies (Meikle, Weed and Tyler, 1975; Pickup, Lowe, Leathan, Rhind, Wright and Downie, 1977; Loo, McGilveray, Jordan, Moffatt and Brien, 1978; Tanner, Bochner, Caffin, Halliday and Powell, 1979) indicated that prednisolone and prednisone appear to exhibit dose-dependent kinetics as might be expected for a compound showing nonlinear protein binding. However, a more recent publication (Al-Habet and Rogers, 1980) concludes that the kinetics of total prednisolone was not dose-dependent. All of the above studies (Meikle et al, 1975; Pickup et al, 1977; Loo et al, 1978; Tanner et al, 1979; Al-Habet and Rogers, 1980) have been carried out using single doses of prednisone or prednisolone; thus, the concentration measurements were not made at steady state. Furthermore, none of the studies have determined whether the interconversion of prednisolone and prednisone is saturable, as we have recently demonstrated in dogs (Frey et al, 1980c). Thus, we undertook to determine unambiguously whether prednisolone exhibits dose-dependent kinetics in man by studying 10 normal individuals at two different steady state prednisolone concentrations (Legler et al, 1982).

Each of the ten volunteers were infused to steady state over a 7 hour period at a low (5.5μg/hr x kg) and a high (64μg/hr x kg) rate with prednisolone. The results of this study are summarized in Table 1.

Table 1 Mean (±SD) parameters and ratio of values obtained during low and high dose prednisolone sodium phosphate 7 hour infusions in ten healthy volunteers

Parameter	Low Dose	High Dose	Ratio High Dose to Low Dose
Infusion Rate (ng/min x kg)	91.8 ± 8.3	1067 ± 115	11.7 ± 1.45
Total Prednisolone Steady-State Concentration (ng/ml)	91 ± 25	437 ± 116	4.9 ± 0.3
Unbound Prednisolone Steady-Stare Concentration (ng/ml)	11 ± 2	103 ± 27	9.5 ± 2.0
Apparent Total Prednisolone Clearance (ml/min x kg)	1.06 ± 0.24	2.54 ± 0.50	2.47 ± 0.29
Apparent Unbound Prednisolone Clearance (ml/min x kg)	8.69 ± 1.58	10.9 ± 2.4	1.29 ± 0.24
Total Prednisone Steady-State Concentration (ng/ml)	13 ± 2	37 ± 4	2.8 ± 0.4
Ratio of Concentrations: Total Prednisolone/ Total Prednisone	6.8 ± 1.3	12.0 ± 3.3	1.8 ± 0.2

Steady state prednisolone levels differed by a factor of 5 when infusion rate was increased approximately 12-fold, indicating a marked increase in the apparent clearance of total prednisolone with increasing dose. The fraction of unbound prednisolone increased from 0.12 ± 0.02 to 0.24 ± 0.02 with increasing dose (Legler et al,1982). Since the increase in the free fraction (2-fold change) was not as great as the increase in apparent clearance of total prednisolone, there was a slight but significant ($p < 0.05$) increase in the apparent clearance of unbound prednisolone (see Table 1).

The interconversion between prednisolone and prednisone appears to approach a maximum prednisone concentration as was previously noted by us in dogs (Frey et al, 1982c). In humans we found this maximum prednisone concentration to be 52 ng/ml when prednisolone is infused. Thus, the ratio of concentrations, prednisolone to prednisone, also increased with increasing prednisolone dose. These results unambiguously indicate that prednisolone exhibits dose and concentration dependent kinetics and that the great majority of the change in kinetics may be attributed to saturable protein binding of prednisolone.

Although some information is available on the pharmacokinetics and bioavailability of prednisone and prednisolone in patients with different disease states, these results may be confounded by the cross reactivity of the assays used with endogenous glucocorticoids as well as by drug metabolites. Two previous studies (Kozower,Veatch and Kaplan,1974; Gambertoglio, Vincenti, Feduska, Birnbaum, Salvatierra and Amend,1980) suggest that the clearance rate of prednisolone may be lower in patients exhibiting cushingoid side effects to glucocorticoid dosing. We investigated the pharmacokinetics of prednisone/prednisolone and the time course of endogenous hydrocortisone in 15 stable renal transplant patients and 12 patients with oral mucocutaneous vesiculoerosive diseases; of the 27 volunteers studied, 14 patients were without cushingoid side effects and 13 had this steroid toxic side effect (Frey et al, 1981a; Frey, Amend, Lozado, Frey and Benet, 1981b). All 27 patients were given their usual prednisone dose orally on one occasion and an equivalent amount of prednisolone intravenously on another occasion. Following dosing, 8 to 14 plasma samples were obtained for the determination of total prednisolone, prednisone and hydrocortisone concentrations by HPLC (Frey et al, 1979) and unbound prednisolone concentrations by equilibrium dialysis. The bioavailability of prednisone, the interconversion of prednisone to prednisolone, the total and unbound prednisolone apparent clearances, the prednisolone binding capacity of albumin and transcortin and the affinity of albumin for prednisolone were not different when the 14 patients without cushingoid side effects were compared with the 13 cushingoid patients. Patients who developed side effects had a higher affinity constant for prednisolone binding to transcortin, more frequently exhibited higher peak hydrocortisone levels and more often had measurable (>10ng/ml) hydrocortisone in the plasma samples collected during the kinetic studies, as compared with those not showing side effects. The data suggest that endogenous hydrocortisone production is not as suppressed in patients with visable cushingoid signs as in noncushingoid patients, and that these is no significant difference in the pharmacokinetics of exogenous glucocorticoids between patients with and without cushingoid side effects.

Our recent work has been related to developing measures of immunosuppression. We first were able to show the expected relation between a pharmacodynamic measure (% MLC inhibition) and plasma levels of total as well as unbound prednisolone in patient plasma following prednisolone or prednisone dosing. Figure 1 depicts the steep hyperbolic concentration-response curve found when % MLC inhibition is plotted vs. unbound prednisolone concentration (Frey et al, 1982). From studies in 12 patients receiving chronic prednisone dosing, we calculated effective concentrations 50% with respect to MLR inhibition for both total and unbound prednisolone following oral and intravenous dosing (Frey et al, 1982). The following mean (±SD) values were found for the EC_{50}(ng/ml): oral dosing - 10.0 ± 5.0 unbound concentration and 86.5 ± 30.9 total concentration; i.v. dosing - 12.4 ± 12.6 bound concentration and 66.3 ± 26.7 total concentration.

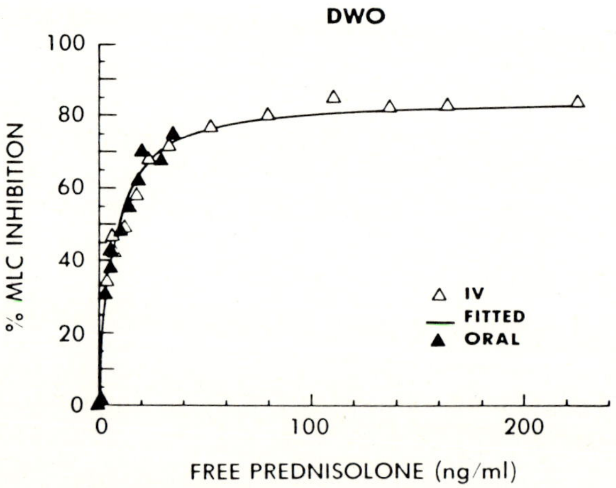

Figure 1 Concentration response curve for free prednisolone in a patient receiving oral prednisone and i.v. prednisolone. The best computer fit line for the intravenous data shown. Both the intravenous and oral data points are plotted (Frey et al, 1982). Reproduced with permission of the publisher.

The EC_{50} values found for total prednisolone following i.v. and oral dosing to the patient population studied here are higher than that found when the inhibition of the MLC is determined following spiking of serial amounts of prednisolone to plasma obtained from a normal volunteer. Tsang and Benet (unpublished results) found an EC_{50} of 29.7 ± 5.7ng/ml for prednisolone in such spiked samples. This difference emphasizes the importance of carrying out the correlation using plasma samples (and preferentially lymphocytes) from the patient population being treated since a variety of suppressive and/or stimulatory humoral factors may be released by treated lymphocyte subpopulations *in vivo*.

We have recently examined the differences between the effects of prednisone, prednisolone and hydrocortisone on the MLR (Tsang, Frey and Benet, 1981). Micro MLCs between normal individuals were cultured in the presence of 15% pooled serum spiked with drug. Cultures were harvested on day 3. As measured by the inhibition of the MLR, predniso-lone is 2 to 2½ times more potent than hydrocortisone (see Fig. 2).

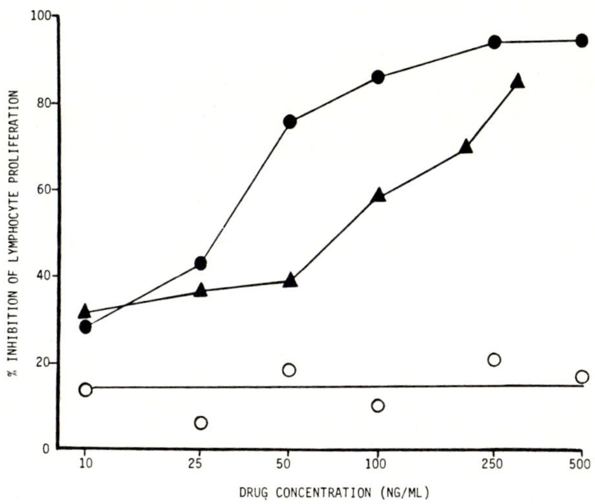

Figure 2 The effect of different concentrations of prednisolone (●), prednisone, (○) and hydrocortisone (▲) on inhibition of the mixed lymphocyte reaction.

Despite their differences in potency, both prednisolone and hydrocorti-sone yield the same maximal inhibition. This maximal inhibition varies with different donor pairs, ranging from 55 to 100%. Prednisone, on the other hand, shows no significant immunosuppressive activity despite the significant slow conversion of prednisone to prednisolone in the MLR by 11-hydroxylation: 28ng/ml prednisolone in a 92ng/ml culture and 44ng/ml in a 460ng/ml culture after 3 days incubation. This finding indicates the importance of the duration and timing of prednisolone's presence in the culture to the overall immunosuppressive activity. The presence of prednisone has no effect on the inhibition due to prednisolone or hydrocortisone.

Since assessment of immunosuppressive capacity in a single plasma sample provides little information concerning the magnitude of immunosuppression over an entire day, we believe that an integrated measure, area under the inhibition curve (AUIC) may be more meaningful. Figure 3 represents the plot of area under the inhibition time curve vs area under the unbound prednisolone concentration time curve following i.v. prednisolone and oral prednisone dosing in the 12 patients discussed above (Frey et al, 1982). We find no simple linear relationship between these values of AUIC and the integrated prednisolone concentrations (AUC). With increasing AUC of prednisolone, the increment of immunosuppression (AUIC) decreases. Provided our model is relevant to the

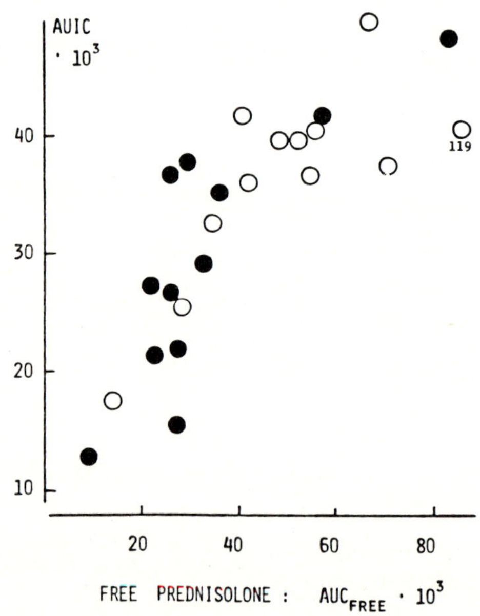

Figure 3 Plot of area under inhibition time curve (AUIC) vs. the area under the unbound prednisolone concentration time curve (AUC_{free}) following oral prednisone (●) and intravenous prednisolone (o) dosing in 12 patients (Frey et al, 1982). Reproduced with permission of the publisher.

clinical situation, doses of prednisone which yield AUC free prednisolone greater than 40,000ng X min/ml will cause little increase in AUIC (see Fig. 3). In most of our subjects, this AUC corresponds to an available prednisone dose of 50mg. Thus, doses of prednisone higher than 50mg may add little to therapeutic efficacy.

To our knowledge, there is no controlled study available at the present which demonstrates that doses higher than 50mg/day add anything to therapeutic efficacy—both for the prevention and treatment of kidney allograft rejections.

We are aware that the MLR inhibition measurement which we have developed is only an intermediate index of immunosuppressive activity. Our long range goal is to extend this correlation between the intermediate index and pharmacokinetics to actual measures of efficacy and toxicity. We are encouraged by our ability to develop a simple, reproducible intermediate measure. In addition, there is rationale for the method chosen since Cochrum and co-workers (1975) did show a correlation of graft survival with a measure of the MLR.

AZATHIOPRINE/6-MERCAPTOPURINE

The biotransformation and biological actions of AZA/6MP have been extensively reviewed (Bach, 1975; Paterson and Tidal, 1975; Elion and Hitchings, 1975; Winkelstein, 1979). AZA's therapeutic and cytotoxic actions are largely attributable to its cleavage to 6MP and subsequent anabolism to thioinosinic acid, and other nucleotides that interfere with nucleic acid synthesis. Therefore, Elion and Hitchings (1975) state that determination of the plasma levels of 6MP or AZA would not have prognostic value with respect to the therapeutic effectiveness or toxicity of these compounds since the biologically active form, thioinosinic acid, occurs within cells. However, in rodents, using extremely large doses of AZA and 6MP, Spreafico and co-workers (Spreafico, Donelli, Bossi, Vecchi, Standen and Garattini, 1973), have shown a good correlation between availability, dose and immunosuppressive activity. In addition, correlations of rosette inhibition activity with radiolabeled levels of AZA and its metabolites have been demonstrated in patients with normal hepatic and renal function (Bach and Dardenne, 1971; Bach and Dardenne, 1972). Therefore, it would appear that some correlations between plasma levels and activity, especially with respect to available dose, may be anticipated.

Specific and sensitive analytical techniques for measuring AZA and 6MP at the levels expected following the usual doses of the drug have only been recently developed. These include direct HPLC assays developed by Ding and Benet (1979), Maddocks (1979a) and Lin, Jessup, Floyd, Wang, Van Buren, Caprioli and Kahan (1980), and a GC/MS method developed by Flobery, Hartvig, Lindstrom, Lonnerholm and Odlind (1981). Pharmacokinetic studies with AZA and 6MP have been carried out in uremic (Odlind, Grefberg, Hartvig, Lindstrom and Lonnerholm, 1982) and kidney transplant patients, (Maddocks, 1979b ; Ding et al, 1980; Lin et al, 1980). The reported pharmacokinetic parameters are summarized in Table 2.

Table 2 Pharmacokinetics of azathioprine and 6-mercaptopurine in uremic and renal transplant patients following azathioprine dosing.

Reference	AZA Measurements (±SD)			6MP Measurements	
	$t_{1/2}$ (min)	Plasma Clearance (ml/min·kg)	Volume of Distribution (L/kg)	$t_{1/2}$ (min)	Availability (%)
Ding et al (1980)	9.7 ± 4.0	57 ± 31	0.81 ± 0.65	63 ± 24	60 ± 31
Lin et al (1980)	11.5 ± 3.0			39 ± 16	
Odlind et al (1982)	40			40	38
Maddocks (1979b)	28			114	

Correlation of AZA/6MP pharmacokinetic data with measures of immunomodulation has not yet been carried out. Correlation of this sort probably will require measurements of intracellular levels of the phosphorylated metabolites of these compounds.

CYCLOPHOSPHAMIDE

Cyclophosphamide (CP) is a potent alkylating agent which has been utilized extensively in recent years, not only in the treatment of cancer, but also as an effective agent in numerous non-malignant, immunologically mediated diseases. Although CP has been used successfully in certain well-defined inflammatory diseases, such as Wegener's granulomatosis (Fauci and Wolff, 1973), and advanced polyarteritis nodosa (Fauci, Koppman and Wolff, 1978), therapy has been mostly empiric due to the difficulty in fully appreciating the pathogenic mechanisms of many of these diseases. Turk and Parker (1979) have reviewed the effect of cyclophosphamide on the immune response, and more recently Stevenson and Fauci (1980) have investigated the differential effects of *in vitro*

CP on human lymphocyte subpopulations involved in B cell activation.

The metabolism and pharmacology of CP have recently been reviewed (Turk and Parker, 1979; Hill, 1975; Cox, Farmer and Jarman, 1976; Domeyer and Sladek, 1980). CP is a prodrug; it must undergo specific metabolism in vivo in order to be active. The key activating step involves hydroxylation to 4-hydroxycyclophosphamide (4-OHCP). This reaction occurs mainly in the liver via the mixed function oxygenase system with NADPH as cofactor. 4-OHCP is thought to be in equilibrium with its open ring tautomer, aldophosphamide (AP). Hydrolysis of AP yields phosphoramide mustard and acrolein. Phosphoramide mustard is believed to be the principal chemotherapeutically active metabolite of CP. It is a potent alkylating agent and is highly cytotoxic, which accounts for the biological activity of CP. Phosphoramide mustard can be further hydrolyzed to yet another cytotoxic metabolite, bis(2-chloroethyl)amine.

4-OHCP and AP can alternatively be oxidized to 4-ketocyclophosphamide and carboxyphosphamide, respectively. These CP metabolites are relatively noncytotoxic with little or no alkylating activity. They account for the major metabolites of CP found in urine. The relative rates at which 4-OHCP/AP is converted to active and inactive metabolites in different cell types may, in part, be the basis for CP's selective toxicity.

Both GC (Juma, Rogers and Trounce, 1979) and GC-MS (Jardine, Fenselau, Appler, Kan, Bundrett and Colvin, 1978) methods have been developed for specific measurement of CP levels in biological fluids. In addition, techniques for the detection of CP's active metabolites have also been recently described (Christian, Chaffee, Hovick and Steele, 1980; Wagner, Heydrich, Jork, Voelcker and Hohorst, 1981). Using these procedures, a number of CP pharmacokinetic studies have been carried out. However, inconsistent results have been reported (Juma et al, 1979; Jardine et al, 1978; Grochow and Colvin, 1979); accurate pharmacokinetic parameters for CP as well as for its metabolites are, therefore, unavailable at present. Considerable work is required before the kinetics of CP and its metabolites are clarified.

CYCLOSPORIN A

Cyclosporin A (Cy-A), a cyclic polypeptide isolated from the fermentation broth of the fungus Trichoderma polysporum, has recently been shown to be a potent immunosuppressive agent. Since its discovery in early 1972, much work has been done in an attempt to elucidate Cy-A's immunosuppressive properties (Borel, 1980; Borel, 1981). However,

Cy-A's mechanism of action remains largely unknown at present. Little information is available on its metabolism and pharmacokinetics, primarily due to difficulties in measuring the drug or its metabolites. Previously developed radioimmunoassay techniques have been found to be technically unsatisfactory and unreliable (Calne, 1980). More recently, a specific RIA (Donatsch, Abisch, Homberger, Traber, Trapp and Voges, 1981) and several HPLC assays (Niederberger, Schaub and Beveridge, 1980; Sawchuk and Cartier, 1981) have been developed. These assays which allow measurement of Cy-A in human blood, plasma and/or urine, allow assessment of drug pharmacokinetic profiles and patient monitoring. Yet, very limited data relating the pharmacokinetic profile of this drug has been reported. Niederberger _et al_ (1980) have studied 2 normal human subjects following a 600mg oral dose of Cy-A. They report half-lives of 5 and 8hr., peak plasma concentrations in the 550-650 ng/ml range and less than 1% of the drug excreted unchanged.

Sawchuk and Cartier (1981) have recently analyzed simultaneous blood and plasma sampled (n=20) from 4 patients on Cy-A. Blood concentrations of Cy-A were found to be significantly higher than those of plasmas, by a ratio of 1.92 (SD ± 0.61), indicating a considerable partition of Cy-A into the RBC.

LEVAMISOLE

Levamisole, a synthetic anthelmintic agent, has been shown to augment both _in vitro_ and _in vivo_ immune responses (Renoux, 1980). Its immunopharmacology has been well reviewed by both Renoux (1980) and Symoens and Rosenthal (1977). Levamisole's immunopotentiating effect varies greatly depending upon time, dose, the genetic background of the host, and the experimental assay used to measure its effect. Furthermore, levamisole is a nonspecific immunostimulator augmenting both lymphocyte effectors and suppressors (Sampson and Lui, 1976).

The metabolism of levamisole has been studied in the rat using labeled material by Janssen Pharmaceutica, Belgium (unpublished studies). Levamisole is extensively metabolized in the liver via several different routes. These pathways include: 1) oxidation of the thiazoline moiety followed by conjugation, 2) oxidation of the imidazoline moiety followed by sulfoxidation, para-hydroxylation and conjugation, 3) para-hydroxylation followed by conjugation, and 4) hydrolysis of the thiazoline moiety to OMPI, a sulphydryl derivative, followed by S-methylation and 2-sulfoxidation. The major metabolite OMPI, (dl-2-oxo-3-(2-mercaptoethyl)5-phenylimidazolidine), is considered to be the active agent.

Janssen Pharmaceutica's unpublished pharmacokinetic studies on levamisole have been reviewed by Adams (1978) and Graziani and De Martin (1977). While most of these studies involved the use of labeled levamisole, polarographic methods were also used to measure the unchanged drug concentrations in tissue (Holbrook and Scales, 1967). Rather limited information is available on the pharmacokinetics of levamisole in man. This is probably due to the lack of convenient and sensitive analytical methods for measuring plasma and tissue levels of levamisole. Recently, HPLC (Marriner, Galbraith and Bogan, 1980; Alvinerie, Galtier and Escoula, 1981) and GC (Woestenborghs, Michielsen and Heykants, 1981) methods have been developed to measure levamisole's plasma and tissue levels. However, more detailed studies on the kinetics of levamisole also require the development of a sensitive assay that can measure the active metabolite, OMPI.

CIMETIDINE

Cimetidine, a histamine H_2 receptor antagonist, is a potent inhibitor of gastric acid secretion and is often used to treat gastric and duodenal ulcerations. Recent clinical and experimental findings suggest that cimetidine may be capable of stimulating the immune system. Cimetidine treatment has been reported to be associated with renal allograft rejection episodes in humans (Primack, 1978), and a significantly shorter graft survival time in dogs (Zammit and Toledo-Pereyra, 1979). Cimetidine therapy has also been found both to restore the skin delayed hypersensitivity response in immunologically impaired patients (Jorizzo, Sams, Jegasothy and Olansky, 1980) and to augment this response in normal subjects (Avella, Madsen, Binder and Askenase, 1978). In addition, cimetidine treatment increases the responsiveness of the patient's lymphocytes to PHA (Robertson, Peden, Saunders, Gibbs, Potts, Brown, Wormsley and Beck, 1979). These effects of cimetidine may be mediated by the blockade of histamine's receptors on regulatory T cells thereby inhibiting histamine's negative feedback action on these cells. *In vitro*, cimetidine augments mitogen-induced lymphocyte blastogenesis (Gifford, Hatfield and Schmidtke, 1980; Palacios and Alarcon-Segovia, 1981). This augmentation effect occurs in the absence of exogenously added histamine and exhibits an unusual dose response relationship. However, these findings, *in vivo* as well as *in vitro*, remain controversial as many investigators have reported conflicting results (Festen, Berden and Koene, 1980; Festen, de Pauw, Smeulders and Wagener, 1981; Doherty and McGeown, 1978; Charpentier and Fries, 1978).

We have examined the effect of cimetidine on the alloantigen-induced lymphocyte proliferation in the mixed lymphocyte culture (MLC) under a variety of conditions. We have found that, over a wide dose range, cimetidine has no significant effect. However, in preliminary experiments, we have seen instances where cimetidine has reduced the inhibitory effect of steroids on the MLC. We have also studied the effect of cimetidine and histamine on the generation of T suppressor (Ts) cells in the primary human MLC and their effect on these cells' suppressive activity on lymphocyte proliferation. Our early work indicates that while histamine increases T_s generation, cimetidine has no effect on Ts generation. However, cimetidine, 10^{-5}M to 10^{-3}M, does decrease the action of Ts cells generated in the presence and absence of histamine. This effect has proven difficult to study because of the large degree of interindividual variability. Cimetidine's effect is most pronounced, completely reversing Ts action, resulting in an increase in lymphocyte proliferation response, when Ts activity is submaximum.

Cimetidine is a particularly interesting drug to study for two reasons. First, in contrast to levamisole, cimetidine appears to selectively inhibit Ts cell function. Secondly, cimetidine has been shown to inhibit microsomal metabolism and therefore impair the elimination of a number of drugs, such as oral anticoagulants, antipyrine, diazapam, phenytoin, theophylline and carbamazepine. The interations of these drugs with cimetidine have been well reviewed by Somogyi and Gugler (1982). Thus, the *in vivo* effects of coadministration of cimetidine and immunosuppressive drugs may yield quantitatively different measures of immunosuppression due to the complicating fact that the immunosuppressive agents may not be cleared from the body as quickly as one expects when cimetidine is present.

The pharmacokinetics of cimetidine have been studied with more accuracy and detail than the other immunoregulating drugs discussed here. Approximately 62 ± 6% of an oral dose is absorbed intact and 77 ± 6% of an i.v. dose is excreted unchanged (Walkenstein, Dubb, Randolph, Westlake, Stote and Intoccia, 1978). Half-life averages 2.1 ± 1.1hr., plasma clearance is 12.3 ± 3.4 ml/min x kg and the volume of distribution is 2.1 ± 1.0 L/kg (Grahnen, von Bahr, Lindstrom and Rosen, 1979). Approximately 19% of the drug is bound to plasma proteins (Somogyi, Rohner and Gugler, 1980).

ACKNOWLEDGEMENTS

Preparation of this manuscript and the studies in the authors' laboratories were supported by National Institutes of Health grants GM 26691 and GM 26551. During the course of this work Ms. Tsang was supported by NIH training grant GM 07175; Dr. Legler by the Deutsche Forschungsgemeinschaft. Drs. Felex J. and Brigitte M. Frey were supported by the Swiss National Foundation for Scientific Research. The authors express their sincere thanks to Ms. Janice Almeida for her aid in preparation of this manuscript.

REFERENCES

ADAMS, J.G. (1978) Pharmacokinetics of levamisole. J. Rheumatol. 5 (Supple. 4), 137.

AL-HABET, S. and ROGERS, H.L. (1980) Pharmacokinetics of intravenous and oral prednisolone. Br. J. Clin. Pharmac. 10, 503.

ALVINERIE, M., GALTIER, P. and ESCOULA, G. (1981) Ion-pair HPLC assay of levamisole in biological fluids. J. Chromatogr. 223, 445.

AVELLA, J., MADSEN, J.E., BINDER, H.J. and ASKENASE, P.W. (1978) Effect of histamine H2-receptor antagonsits on delayed hypersensitivity. Lancet 1, 624.

BACH, J.F. (1975) The Mode of Action of Immunosuppressive Agents. North Holland Publ., Amsterdam.

BACH, J.F. and DARDENNE, M. (1971) The metabolism of azathioprine in renal failure. Transplantation 12, 253.

BACH, J.F. and DARDEENE, M. (1972) Serum immunosuppressive activity of azathioprine in normal subjects and patients with liver diseases. Proc. Roy. Soc. Med. 65, 260.

BENET, L.Z., FREY, B.M., DING, T.L. and FREY, F.J. (1981) The pharmacokinetics of immunoregulating drugs - immunopharmacokinetics. In: Advances in Immunopharmacology (eds. Hadden, J., Chedid, L., Mullen, P. and Spreafico, F.) Pergamon Press, Oxford. pp. 29-36.

BOREL, J.F. (1980) Essentials of cyclosporin A. Trends Pharmacol Sci. 2, 146.

BOREL, J.F. (1981) Cyclosporin-A: Present experimental status. Transplantation Proc. 13, 344.

CALNE, R.Y. (1980) Cyclosporin. Nephron 26, 57.

CHARPENTIER, B. and FRIES, D. (1978) Cimetidine and renal-allograft rejection. Lancet 1, 1265.

CHRISTIAN, R.A., CHAFFEE, S.K., HOVICK, C.J. and STEELE, W.J. (1980) A stable colorimetric assay for cyclophosphamide and its aldylating metabolites based on the alkylation of 4-(4^1-nitrobenzyl)-pyridine. Life Sci. 27, 2595.

COCHRUM, K.C., SALVATIERRA, O., PERKINS, H.A. and BELZER, F.O. (1975) MLC testing in renal transplantation. Transplant Proc. 7, (Suppl. 1), 659.

COX, P.J., FARMER, P.B. and JARMAN, M. (eds.) (1976) Symposium on the Metabolism and Mechanisms of Action of Cyclophosphamide. Cancer Treat. Reports 60, 299.

DING, T.L. and BENET, L.Z. (1979) Determination of 6-mercaptopurine and azathioprine in plasma by high-performance liquid chromatography. J. Chromatogr. 163, 281.

DING, T.L., GAMBERTOGLIO, J.G., AMEND, W.J.C., BIRNBAUM, J. and BENET, L.Z. (1980) Azathioprine (AZA) bioavailability and pharmacokinetics in kidney transplant patients. Clin. Pharmac. Therap. 27, 250.

DOHERTY, C.C. and McGEOWN, M.G. (1978) Cimetidine and renal-allograft rejection. Lancet 1, 1048.

DOMEYER, B.E. and SLADEK, N.E. (1980) Metabolism of 4-hydroxycyclophosphamide/aldophosphamide in vitro. Biochem. Pharmac. 29, 2903.

DONATSCH, P., ABISCH, E., HOMBERGER, M., TRABER, R., TRAPP, M. and VOGES, R. (1981) A radioimmunoassay to measure cyclosporin A in plasma and serum samples. J. Immunoassay 2, 19.

ELION, G.B. and HITCHINGS, G.H. (1975) Azathioprine. In: Antineoplastic and Immunosuppressive Agents (eds. Sartorelli, A.C. and John, D.G.) part II, Springer-Verleg, Berlin. pp. 404-425.

FAUCI, A.S. (1979) Mechanisms of the immunosuppressive and anti-inflammatory effects of glucocorticosteroids. J. Immunopharmac. 1, 1.

FAUCI, A.S., DALE, D.C. and BALOW, J.E. (1976) Glucocorticosteroid therapy: mechanisms of action and clinical considerations. Ann. Intern. Med. 84, 304.

FAUCI, A.S., KOPPMAN, J.L. and WOLFF, S.M. (1978) Cyclophosphamide-induced remissions in advanced ployarteritis nodosa. Am. J. Med. 64, 890.

FAUCI, A.S. and WOLFF, S.M. (1973) Wegener's granulomatosis: studies in eighteen patients and a review of the literature. Medicine 52, 535.

FESTEN, H.P.M., BERDEN, J.H.M. and KOENE, R.A.P. (1980) Cimetidine does not accelerate skin graft rejection in mice. Clin. Exp. Immun. 40, 193.

FESTEN, H.P.M., dePAUW, B.E., SMEULDERS, J. and WAGENER, D.J.Th. (1981) Cimetidine does not influence immunological parameters in man. Clin. Immun. and Immunopath. 21, 33.

FLOBERY, S., HARTVIG, P., LINDSTROM, B., LONNERHOLM, G. and ODLIND, B. (1981) Extractive alkylation of plasma samples of 6-mercaptopurine and determination by gas chromatography mass spectrometry. J. Chromatogr. 225, 73.

FREY, B.M., FREY, F.J. and BENET, L.Z. (1979) Liquid chromatographic measurement of endogenous and exogenous glucocorticoids in plasma. Clin. Chem. 25, 1944.

FREY, B.M., FREY, F.J., BENET, L.Z. and COCHRUM. K.C. (1980a) Modification of the mixed lymphocyte reaction for pharmacokinetic assessment of immunosuppressive activity in human plasma. Int. J. Immunopharmac. 2, 129.

FREY, B.M., FREY, F.J., COCHRUM, K.C. and BENET, L.Z. (1980b) Induction kinetics of human suppressor cells in the mixed lymphocyte reaction and influence of prednisolone on their genesis. Cellular Immunol. 56, 225.

FREY, B.M., FREY, F.J., HOLFORD, N.K.G., LOZADA, F. and BENET, L.Z. (1982) Prednisolone pharmacodynamics assessed by inhibition of the mixed lymphocyte reaction. Transplantation 33, 578.

FREY, F.J., AMEND, Jr., W.J.C., LOZADA, F., FREY, B.M. and BENET, L.Z. (1981b) Endogenous hydrocortisone, a possible factor contributing to the genesis of cushingoid habitus in patients on prednisone. J. Clin. Endocrinol. Metab. 53, 1076.

FREY, F.J., AMEND, W.J.C., LOZADA, F., FREY, B.M., HOLFORD, N.H.G. and BENET, L.Z. (1981a) Pharmacokinetics of prednisolone and endogenous hydrocortisone levels in cushingoid and noncushingoid patients. Eur. J. Clin. Pharmac. 21, 235.

FREY, F.J., FREY, B.M., GREITHER, A. and BENET, L.Z. (1980c) Prednisolone clearance at steady state in dogs. J. Pharmac. Exp. Ther. 215, 287.

GAMBERTOGLIO, J.G., AMEND, W.J.C. and BENET, L.Z. (1980) Pharmacokinetics and bioavailability of prednisone and prednisolone in healthy volunteers and patients: a review. J. Pharmacokinet. Biopharm. 8, 1.

GAMBERTOGLIO, J., VINCENTI, F., FEDUSKA, N., BIRNBAUM, J., SALVATIERRA, O. and AMEND, W. (1980) Prednisolone disposition in cushingoid and noncushingoid kidney transplant patients. J. Clin. Endocrinol. Metab. 51, 561.

GIFFORD, R.R.M., HATFIELD, S.M. and SCHMIDTKE, J.R. (1980) Cimetidine-induced augmentation of human lymphocyte blastogenesis by mitogen, bacterial antigen, and alloantigen. Transplantation 29, 143.

GRAHNEN, A., von BAHR, C., LINDSTROM, B. and ROSEN, A. (1979). Bioavailability and pharmacokinetics of cimetidine. Eur. J. Clin. Pharmac., 16, 335.

GRAZIANI, G. and De MARTIN, G.L. (1977) Pharmacokinetic studies on levamisole. Drugs Exptl. Clin. Res. 2, 221.

GROCHOW, L.B. and COLVIN, M. (1979) Clinical pharmacokinetics of cyclophosphamide. Clin. Pharmacokinet. 4, 380.

HILL, D.L. (1975) A Review of Cyclophosphamide Charles C. Thomas, Springfield, IL.

HOLBROOK, A. and SCALES, B. (1967) Polarographic determination of tetramisole hydrochloride in extracts of animal tissue. Analyt. Biochem. 18, 46.

ILFELD, D.N., KRAKAUER, R.S. and BLAESE, R.M. (1977) Suppression of the human autologous mixed lymphocyte reaction by physiologic concentrations of hydrocortisone. J. Immun. 119, 428.

JARDINE, I., FENSELAU, C., APPLER, M., KAN, M.N., BUNDRETT, R.B. and COLVIN, M. (1978) Quantitation by gas chromatography-chemical ionization mass spectrometry of cyclophosphamide, phosphoramide mustard, and nornitrogen mustard in the plasma and urine of patients receiving cyclophosphamide therapy. Cancer Res. 38, 408.

JORIZZO, J.L., SAMS, W.M., JEGASOTHY, B.V. and OLANSKY, A.J. (1980) Cimetidine as an immunomodulator: chronic mucocutaneous candidiasis as a model. Annals of Internal Medicine 92, (Part 1), 192.

JUMA, F.D., ROGERS, H.J. and TROUNCE, J.R. (1979) Pharmacokinetics of cyclophosphamide and alkylating activity in man after intravenous and oral administration. Br. J. Clin. Pharmac. 8, 209.

KOZOWER, M., VEATCH, L. and KAPLAN, M.M. (1974) Decreased clearance of prednisolone, a factor in the development of corticosteroid side effecrs. J. Clin. Endocrinol. Metab. 38, 407.

LEGLER, U.F., FREY, F.J. and BENET, L.Z. (1982) Prednisolone clearance at steady state in man. J. Clin. Endocrinol. Metab. 55, in press, Oct. 1982.

LIN, S.N., JESSUP, K., FLOYD, M., WANG, T.P.F., van BUREN, C.T., CAPRIOLI, R.M. and KAHAN, B.D. (1980) Quantitation of plasma azathioprine and 6-mercaptopurine levels in renal transplant patients. Transplantation 29, 290.

LOO, J.C.K., McGILVERAY, I.J., JORDAN, N., MOFFATT, J. and BRIEN, R. (1978) Dose-dependent pharmacokinetics of prednisone and prednisolone in man. J. Pharm. Pharmacol. 30, 736.

MADDOCKS, J.L. (1979a) Assay of azathioprine, 6-mercaptopurine and a novel thiopurine metabolite in human plasma. Br. J. Clin. Pharmac. 8, 273.

MADDOCKS, J.L. (1979b) Progress in Immunosuppression. In: Topics in Therapeutics, Vol. 5 (eds. Davies, D.M. and Rawlins, M.D.) G.K. Hall, Boston. pp. 33-44.

MARRINER, S., GALBRAITH, E.A. and BOGAN, J.A. (1980) Determination of the anthelmintic levamisole in plasma and GI fluids by HPLC. Analyst. 105, 993.

MEIKLE, A.W., WEED, J.A. and TYPER, F.H. (1975) Kinetics and interconversion of prednisolone and prednisone studied with new radioimmunoassays. J. Clin. Endocrinol. Metab. 41, 717.

NIEDERBERGER, W., SCHAUB, P. and BEVERIDGE, T. (1980) High-performance liquid chromatographic determination of cyclosporin A in human plasma and urine. J. Chromatogr. 182, 454.

ODLIND, B., GREFBERG, N., HARTVIG, P., LINDSTROM, B. and LONNERHOLM, G. (1982) Pharmacokinetics of azathioprine and 6-mercaptopurine: methodological aspects and preliminary results in uremic patients. Scand. J. Nephrol. Urol., (in press).

PALACIOS, R. and ALARCON-SEGOVIA, D. (1981) Cimetidine abrogates suppressor T cell function in vitro. Immunology Letters 3, 33.

PATERSON, A.R.P. and TIDD, D.M. (1975) 6-Thiopurines. In: Antineoplastic and Immunosuppressive Agents (eds. Sartolli, A.C. and Johns, D.G.), Springer-Verlag, Berlin. pp. 384-403.

PICKUP, M.E. (1979) Clinical pharmacokinetics of prednisone and prednisolone. Clin. Pharmacokinet. 4, 111.

PICKUP, M.E., LOWE, J.R., LEATHAN, P.A., RHIND, V.M., WRIGHT, V. and DOWNIE, W.W. (1977) Dose-dependent pharmacokinetics of prednisolone. Eur. J. Clin. Pharmac. 12, 213.

PRIMACK, W.A. (1978) Cimetidine and renal-allograft rejection. Lancet 1, 824.

RENOUX, G. (1980) The general immunopharmacology of levamisole. Drugs 19, 89.

ROBERTSON, A.J., PEDEN, N.R., SAUNDERS, J.H.B., GIBBS, J.H., POTTS, R.C., BROWN, R.A., WORMSLEY, K.G. and BECK, J.S. (1979) Cimetidine and the immune response. Lancet 2, 420.

SAMPSON, D. and LUI, A. (1976) The effect of levamisole on cell-mediated immunity and suppressor cell function. Cancer Res. 36, 952.

SAWCHUK, R.J. and CARTIER, L.L. (1981) Liquid-chromatographic determination of cyclosporin A in blood and plasma. Clin. Chem. 27, 1368.

SOMOGYI, A. and GUGLER, R. (1982) Drug interactions with cimetidine. Clin. Pharmacokinet. 7, 23.

SOMOGYI, A., ROHNER, H.G., and GUGLER, R. (1980) Pharmacokinetics and bioavailability of cimetidine in gastric and duodenal ulcer patients. Clin. Pharmacokinet. 5, 84.

SPREAFICO, F., DONELLI, M.G., BOSSI, A., VECCHI, A., STANDEN, S. and GARATTINI, S. (1973) Immunodepressant activity and 6-mercaptopurine levels after administration of 6-mercaptopurine and azathioprine. Transplantation 16, 269.

STEVENSON, H.C. and FAUCI, A.S. (1980) Activation of human β lymphocytes XII. Differential effects of in vitro cyclophosphamide on human lymphocyte subpopulations involved in β-cell activation. Immunology 39, 391.

SYMOENS, J. and ROSENTHAL, M. (1977) Levamisole in the modulation of the immune response: the current experimental and clinical state. J. Reticuloendothel. Soc. 21, 175.

TANNER, A., BOCHNER, F., CAFFIN, J., HALLIDAY, J. and POWELL, L. (1979) Dose-dependent prednisolone kinetics. Clin. Pharmacol. Ther. 25, 571.

TSANG, S.Y., FREY, B.M. and BENET, L.Z. (1981) Effects of corticosteroids on the in vitro proliferative response of human lymphocytes to allogeneic cells. Abstracts of APhA Academy of Pharmaceutical Sciences 11, (2), 143.

TURK, J.L. and PARKER, D. (1979) The effect of cyclophosphamide on the immune response. J. Immunopharmacol. 1, 127.

WAGNER, T., HEYDRICH, D., JORK, T., VOELCKER, G. and HOHORST, H.J. (1981) Comparative study on human pharmacokinetics of activated ifostamide and cyclophosphamide by a modified fluorometric test. J. Cancer Res. Clin. Oncol., 100, 95.

WALKENSTEIN, S.S., DUBB, J.W., RANDOLPH, W.C., WESTLAKE, W.J., STOTE, R.M. and INTOCCIA, A.P. (1978) Bioavailability of cimetidine in man. Gastroenterology 74, 360.

WINKELSTEIN, A. (1979) The effects of azathioprine and 6 MP on immunity. J. Immunopharmacol. 1, 429.

WOESTENBORGHS, R., MICHIELSEN, L. and HEYKANTS, J. (1981) Determination of levamisole in plasma and animal tissues by GC with thermionic specific detection. J. Chromatogr. 224, 25.

ZAMMIT, M. and TOLEDO-PEREYRA (1979) Cimetidine for kidney transplantation: experimental observations. Surgery 86, 611.

THE HUMORAL IMMUNOTOXICOLOGICAL EFFECTS OF PHENYTOIN—AN ANTICONVULSANT DRUG WITH NONLINEAR PHARMACOKINETICS

Peter W. Mullen[1] and Mary L.S. Queiroz[2]

[1]Kemic Bioresearch Laboratories Limited
Kentville, Nova Scotia, Canada, B4N 4H8

[2]Department of Pharmacology, University of Manchester, Manchester, U.K., M13 9PT

Over the past two decades, a number of reports have provided evidence that phenytoin (diphenylhydantoin) and other widely-used anti-epileptic drugs may alter immune function (MacKinney and Booker, 1972; Sorrell and Forbes, 1975; Seager, Jamison, Wilson, Hayward and Soothill, 1975; Levo, Markowitz and Trainin, 1975; Aarli, 1976; Bluming, Homer and Khiroya, 1976; Fontana, Sauter, Grob and Joller, 1976; Fossan, 1977; Hornby and Mullen, 1977; Queiroz and Mullen, 1980; Thatcher, Wan, Swindell, Wilkinson and Crowther, 1982; Dosch, Jason and Gelfand, 1982; Gilhus, Aarli and Thorsby, 1982; Gilhus, 1983).

In mice Kruger (1970) observed that phenytoin produced distinct histological changes in lymphoid tissues after a two month period of oral administration. After daily subcutaneous injections for two weeks, Levo et al (1975) found that phenytoin (500µg per mouse) did not affect spleen cell responsiveness to concanavalin A; humoral immunity, as indicated by the Jerne plaque-forming cell assay, was much reduced, however. (Interestingly, these workers also noted fewer urethane-induced lung adenomas in phenytoin treated animals, presumably due to diminished "blocking factor" production.)

In humans, lymphopenia may occur at high serum phenytoin concentrations (MacKinney and Booker, 1972) and, in certain patients, especially those possessing the HLA-A_2 antigen, both serum and salivary IgA levels may be decreased by phenytoin treatment (Seager et al, 1975; Aarli, 1976; Fontana et al, 1976; Gilhus et al, 1982). Moreover, a few patients receiving phenytoin have developed reversible lymphoproliferative disorders and/or allergic reactions (Grams, Neal and Conrad, 1968; Lapes, Vivacqua and Antoniades, 1976; Dosch et al, 1982) which, at least in one case, may have been associated with malfunctioning suppressor T-lymphocytes (Dosch et al, 1982).

NATO ASI Series, Vol. G2
Immunotoxicology. Edited by P. W. Mullen

In vitro treatment of human lymphocytes reduces the percentage of cells which form "E-rosettes" with sheep erythrocytes (Hornby and Mullen, 1977; Gilhus, 1983).

RECENT FINDINGS IN ANIMALS

In Vitro Studies:

Since phenytoin undergoes extensive biotransformation *in vivo*, we (Queiroz and Mullen, 1980) undertook to investigate the comparative effects of this drug and its principal metabolite, 5-(p-hydroxyphenyl)-5-phenylhydantoin (HPPH) on *in vitro* immune responses.

Approximately seventy percent of administered phenytoin may be recovered in the urine as the glucuronide conjugate of the HPPH biotransformation product (Maynert, 1960).

Spleen cells from mice which had been immunized with sheep erythrocytes (SRBC) were incubated for 75 minutes with various concentrations of phenytoin or HPPH in Medium 199. The treated cells were then subjected to the direct plaque-forming cell assay of Jerne, Nordin and Henry (1963).

As seen in Table I, SRBC-sensitized spleen cells incubated with phenytoin at concentrations of 10, 20 and 50 mg/L produced increased numbers of plaques in the Jerne assay. In contrast, in concomitant experiments using the same spleen cell suspensions, HPPH, even at the higher 50 mg/L concentration, had no effect in this assay relative to control cells not preincubated with drug. Cell viability as determined by a trypan blue exclusion procedure was unaffected by the concentrations of phenytoin or HPPH used in these experiments.

Table I. *In vitro* effects of phenytoin and its major hydroxy-metabolite (HPPH) on the number of antibody secreting spleen cells (plaque forming cells, PFC) per culture from SRBC-immunized mice.

Drug*	Concentration (mg/L)	Percentage Change in PFCs Relative to Control	Statistical Significance[+]
Phenytoin	50	+ 53.5%	$p < 0.001$
Phenytoin	20	+ 61.4%	$p < 0.001$
Phenytoin	10	+ 35.0%	$p < 0.01$
HPPH	50	+ 3.4%	N.S.

* Spleen cells were incubated with the compound *in vitro* for 75 minutes prior to the determination of PFC. Control cells were incubated in medium containing vehicle only.

[+] Determined by a two-tailed paired t-test (drug treated versus control cell suspensions; n = 6-7 experiments).

In Vivo Studies:

Phenytoin and HPPH in doses of 2, 10, 20 and 50 mg/kg (or vehicle only in the case of control groups) were administered (i.p.) on alternate days to different groups of mice for periods of one, three and seven weeks. Three days prior to the last dose of phenytoin or HPPH, each mouse was immunized with SRBCs (0.2ml of 10% SRBC, i.p.). Four days after immunization the animals were killed and their spleen plaque forming cell capacity was determined using the Jerne assay procedure (Queiroz and Mullen, 1980).

Alternate day treatment with these compounds for one week had no significant effect on the number of plaque forming cells (PFCs). However, a dose-related decrease in the number of PFCs was observed relative to control animals after the three week (Figure 1) and seven week (data not shown) treatment periods.

Specifically, both phenytoin and HPPH at the 10 and 20mg/kg and 10, 20 and 50mg/kg alternate day dosing schedules, respectively, induced significant reductions in the number of PFCs (Queiroz and Mullen, 1980; Mullen and Queiroz, 1983). A significant decrease in spleen weights however, occurred only with the highest dose (i.e. 50mg/kg) of HPPH.

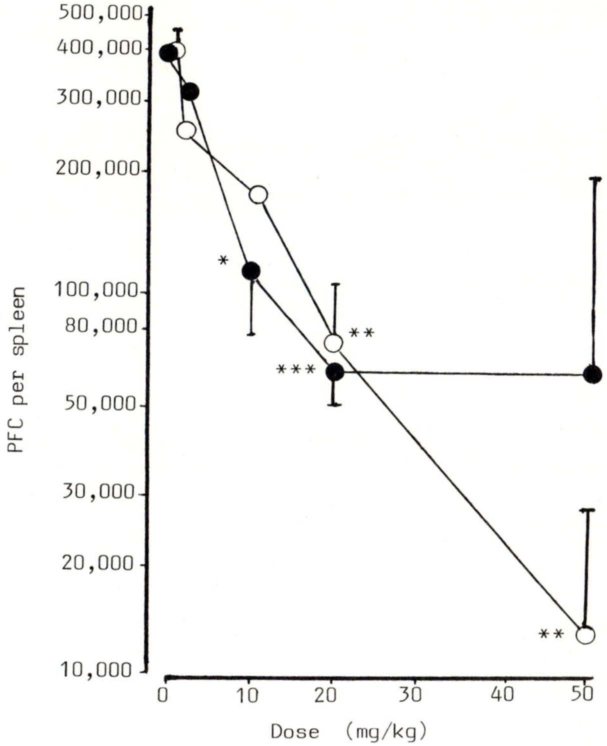

Figure 1 The number of direct (mainly IgM) plaque forming cells per spleen (PFC) after alternate day treatment (i.p.) with phenytoin (-●-) or HPPH (-○-) for three weeks. Each point represents the mean (n = 7) ± S.E.M. (*p = 0.02; ** p ≤ 0.005; *** p ≤ 0.0005) as determined by a 2 tailed "t-test".

The variability observed with the highest dosing schedule (50mg/kg on alternate days) of phenytoin in the three (Figure 1) and seven week experiments is in marked contrast to the findings obtained with HPPH. Moreover, these *in vivo* effects on humoral immunity produced by phenytoin and its HPPH metabolite differ from those observed after *in vitro* preincubation of sensitized spleenocytes with these compounds prior to the plaque assay. As described above, in the *in vitro* experiments phenytoin enhanced, while HPPH had no effect on, PFC numbers, whereas *in vivo*, both agents were found to reduce the number of antibody producing cells (except for the inconsistent effect of phenytoin at the 50mg/kg dose).

To account for their different effects *in vitro* and *in vivo* it could be postulated that both phenytoin and its major metabolite, HPPH, undergo additional biotransformation to a common immunosuppressive product. On the basis of this assumption, the inconsistent effects on humoral immunity of phenytoin at very high doses (ca. 50mg/kg) *in vivo* may be explained if one considers the unique pharmacokinetic characteristics of this drug.

A PHARMACOKINETIC INTERPRETATION OF PHENYTOIN'S EFFECTS ON HUMORAL IMMUNITY

Interestingly, with respect to the *in vivo* animal studies discussed above, it should be pointed out that, with the exception of the highest dose employed, the quantities of phenytoin administered, when considered on an average daily basis are equivalent to 1, 5, 10 and 25 mg/kg/day, approximating those doses used therapeutically in the treatment of human epilepsy. Also, it is now known that at very high doses of phenytoin, the concentration ratio of unchanged drug to metabolite(s) in the body is much greater than at lower doses, due to the readily saturable nature of the biotransformation kinetics of this drug (Gerber and Arnold, 1969; Mawer, Mullen, Rodgers, Robins and Lucas, 1974; Mullen, 1978; Mullen and Foster, 1979).

As a result of phenytoin's "dose-dependent" or Michaelis-Menten pharmacokinetics in various species, including the mouse (Gerber and Arnold, 1969), a nonlinear relationship occurs between the serum drug concentration in the steady-state and the dose similar to that shown in Figure 2 (Mawer *et al*, 1974; Mullen and Foster, 1979). In other words, the steady-state serum phenytoin concentration observed upon repeated dosing will markedly and disproportionately increase as the dose is increased.

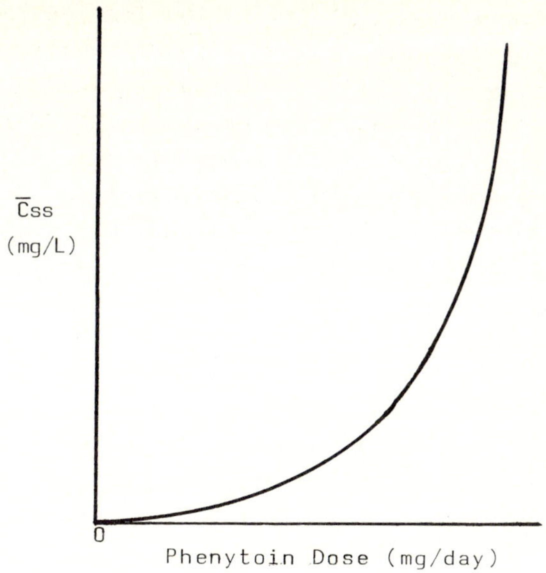

Figure 2 Typical relationship between steady-state serum phenytoin concentration $\bar{C}ss$ and daily dose (Mullen and Foster, 1979).

Phenytoin *per se* enhances humoral immunity as indicated by the *in vitro* studies. However, assuming that it is metabolized to a product which is immunosuppressive, then the large increase in levels of unchanged phenytoin relative to its metabolite would, at high doses (e.g. 50 mg phenytoin/kg), tend to shift the observed (net) immunological effect towards immune enhancement.

CONCLUDING COMMENTS

Phenytoin *in vivo* demonstrably suppresses humoral immunity at relatively low doses. However, given the possibility that phenytoin *per se* actually possesses the capacity to enhance humoral immune responses, it is essential to realize that conceivably there are a range of possible effects on the immune system depending upon the dose and pharmacokinetic characteristics of this drug in a particular individual patient. The need for caution when extrapolating from *in vitro* experiments to the *in vivo* situation is made obvious by the work described here with phenytoin and by others studying different agents (Wess and

Archer, 1982).

To verify the assumptions made above it will be necessary to design further experiments both in vitro and in vivo to determine the comparative immune effects of phenytoin and its various biotransformation products (including the glucuronide conjugate of HPPH). Certainly the limited findings with phenytoin discussed above serve, at the very least, to emphasize the importance of considering biotransformation and pharmacokinetic principles when interpreting the results of immunopharmacological research.

REFERENCES

AARLI, J.A. (1976) Drug-induced IgA deficiency in epileptic patients. Arch. Neurol. 33, 296.

BLUMING, A., HOMER, S. and KHIROYA, R. (1976) Selective diphenylhydantoin-induced suppression of lymphocyte reactivity in vitro. J. Lab. Clin. Med. 88, 417.

DOSCH, H.M., JASON, J. and GELFAND, E.W. (1982) Transient antibody deficiency and abnormal T-suppressor cells induced by phenytoin. New Eng. J. Med. 306, 406.

FONTANA, A., SAUTER, R., GROB, P.J. and JOLLER, H. (1976) IgA deficiency, epilepsy and hydantoin medication. Lancet 2, 228.

FOSSAN, G.O. (1977) Effect of phenytoin on the immune response in rabbits. Int. Archs. Allergy Appl. Immun. 54, 338.

GAMS, R.A., NEAL, J.A. and CONRAD, F.G. (1968) Hydantoin induced pseudolymphoma. Ann. Intern. Med. 69, 557.

GERBER, N. and ARNOLD, K. (1969) Studies on the metabolism of diphenylhydantoin in mice. J. Pharmac. Exp. Ther. 167, 77.

GILHUS, N.E., AARLI, J.A. and THORSBY, E. (1982) HLA antigens in epileptic patients with drug-induced immunodeficiency. Int. J. Immunopharmac. 4, 517.

GILHUS, N.E. (1983) The in vitro effect of phenytoin and carbamazepine on subpopulations of human blood mononuclear cells. Int. J. Immunopharmac. 5, 283.

HORNBY, C. and MULLEN, P.W. (1977) The effects of phenytoin on T-lymphocyte enumeration. Br. J. Pharmac. 61, 454P.

JERNE, N.K., NORDIN, A.A. and HENRY, C. (1963) The agar plaque technique for recognizing antibody producing cells. p. 109 In: Cell-bound Antibodies (eds. Amos, H. and Kaprowski, H.) Wistar Institute Press, Philadelphi

KRUGER, G. (1970) Effect of Dilantin in mice. I. Changes in the lymphoreticular tissue after acute exposure. Virchows Arch. Path. Anat. Physiol. 349, 297.

LAPES, M.J., VIVACQUE, R.J. and ANTONIADES, K. (1976) Immunoblastic lymphadenopathy associated with phenytoin (diphenylhydantoin). Lancet 1, 198.

LEVO, Y., MARKOWITZ, O. and TRAININ, N. (1975) Hydantoin immunosuppression and carcinogenesis. Clin. Exp. Immun. 19, 521.

MACKINNEY, A.A. and BOOKER, H.E. (1972) Diphenylhydantoin effects on human lymphocytes in vitro and in vivo. Arch. Intern. Med. 129, 988.

MAWER, G.E., MULLEN, P.W., RODGERS, M., ROBINS, A.G. and LUCAS, S.B. (1974) Phenytoin dose adjustment in epileptic patients. Br. J. Clin. Pharmac. 1, 163.

MAYNERT, E.W. (1960) The metabolic fate of diphenylhydantoin in the dog, rat and man. J. Pharmac. Exp. Ther. 130, 275.

MULLEN, P.W. (1978) Optimal phenytoin therapy: A new technique for individualizing dosage. Clin. Pharmacol. Ther. 23, 228.

MULLEN, P.W. and FOSTER, R.W. (1979) Comparative evaluation of six techniques for determining the Michaelis-Menten parameters relating phenytoin dose and steady-state serum concentrations. J. Pharm. Pharmac. 31, 100.

MULLEN, P.W. and QUEIROZ, M.L.S. (1983) Phenytoin and humoral immunity: background and a pharmacokinetic interpretation of recent findings. p. 3. In: Advances in Immunopharmacology 2, (eds. Hadden, J., Chedid, L., Dukor, P., Spreafico, F. and Willoughby, D.) Pergamon Press, U.K.

QUEIROZ, M.L.S. and MULLEN, P.W. (1980) The effects of phenytoin, 5-(para-hydroxyphenyl)-5-phenylhydantoin and valproic acid on humoral immunity in mice. Int. J. Immunopharmac. 2, 224.

SEAGER, J., JAMISON, D.L., WILSON, J., HAYWARD, A.R. and SOOTHILL, J.F. (1975) IgA deficiency, epilepsy, and phenytoin treatment. Lancet 2, 632.

SORRELL, T.C. and I.J. FORBES (1975) Depression of immune competence by phenytoin and carbamazepine. Clin. Exp. Immunol. 20, 273.

THATCHER, N., WAN, H.H., SWINDELL, R., WILKINSON, P.M. and CROWTHER, D. (1982) Effects of diphenylhydantoin on killer cell activity and other immunological functions. Int. J. Immunopharmac. 4, 167.

WESS, J.A. and ARCHER, D.L. (1982) Disparate in vivo and in vitro immunomodulatory activities of rhodamine B. Fd. Chem. Toxic. 20, 9.

VIRAL INFECTION AND XENOBIOTIC METABOLISM

Kenneth W. Renton and Gurmit Singh
Department of Pharmacology
Dalhousie University
Halifax, Nova Scotia
B3H 4H7 Canada

The rate of drug biotransformation in the liver plays a major role in determining the intensity and duration of action of a large number of commonly used drugs, chemicals and carcinogens (Peterson and Holtzman, 1980). Most drugs and chemicals would be retained in the body for indefinite periods if they were not metabolized to more polar products which can be readily excreted in the urine or bile. A major portion of drug and chemical biotransformation is carried out by an enzyme system with a broad substrate specificity commonly called "mixed-function oxidase" with cytochrome P-450 as its central component and which is located in the endoplasmic reticulum of the hepatocyte. The steady state level of cytochrome P-450 and the capacity of the liver to metabolize drugs can be altered by many endogenous chemicals, physiological factors and pathological states. Certain species of cytochrome P-450 are induced by agents such as phenobarbital and other species of the hemoprotein by chemicals related to polycyclic hydrocarbons. Inhibition or destruction of the enzyme system has been reported for many different chemicals. In practical terms the therapy of disease with drugs which depend on cytochrome P-450 for biotransformation and elimination is often complicated by changes in cytochrome P-450 steady state levels. Such changes in drug biotransformation account for a large number of observed drug reactions and interactions. When individuals are given drugs or are exposed to chemicals repeatedly the compounds may accumulate and produce toxic results if the cytochrome P-450 system is depressed. On the other hand, if the cytochrome P-450 system is induced the duration of action of drugs is diminished and often little therapeutic benefit occurs.

In addition to the large number of factors which can alter rates of drug biotransformation, it has recently been recognized that changes in drug metabolism occur during infections or following the administration of immuno-active agents. This interaction between host defense mechanisms and drug elimination is an important consideration when drugs are used in an infected individual.

A large number of non-specific immunostimulants can depress hepatic microsomal drug biotransformation and decrease the capacity of the liver

NATO ASI Series, Vol. G2
Immunotoxicology. Edited by P. W. Mullen

to eliminate drugs (Renton 1982). These agents are listed in Table 1.

Table 1 Immuno-modulators which depress cytochrome P-450 mediated drug formation biotransformation

B.pertussis	Colloidal Carbon
C.parvum	Dextran
M.butyricum	Dextran SO_4
BCG	Latex beads
Freunds Adjuvant	Trypan Blue
E.coli endotoxin	Maleic divinylether copolymers
Zymosan	Tilorone
Statolon	Poly rI.rC
Quinacrine	Interferon
	Viral infection

Because these agents have a wide variety of common properties it has been difficult to determine exactly which mechanisms are involved in depressing cytochrome P-450 and drug metabolism. In recent work using *B. pertussis*, Williams, Winters, Lowitt and Szentivanji (1981) have demonstrated that at least two components of this agent can lower cytochrome P-450 and that the T cell mediated immune system is involved in the action of the heat sensitive component. On the other hand, *C.parvum* (Soyka, Stephens, MacPherson and Foster, 1979) may lower cytochrome P-450 by a third mechanism which involves macrophage function. As will be discussed later many of these agents also induce interferon which is also implicated in lowering drug metabolism. Overall it is very unlikely that a single mechanism can explain the action of all of the agents listed in Table 1.

Although in 1976 we proposed that interferon could depress cytochrome P-450 and related drug biotransformation (Renton and Mannering, 1976) it is only recently that definite proof for such an affect has been established. Initially a large number of interferon inducers were shown to depress cytochrome P-450 and the temporal relationship between the appearance of interferon following the administration of poly rI.rC and the depression of cytochrome P-450 strongly suggested that interferon was responsible for this effect (Fig. 1).

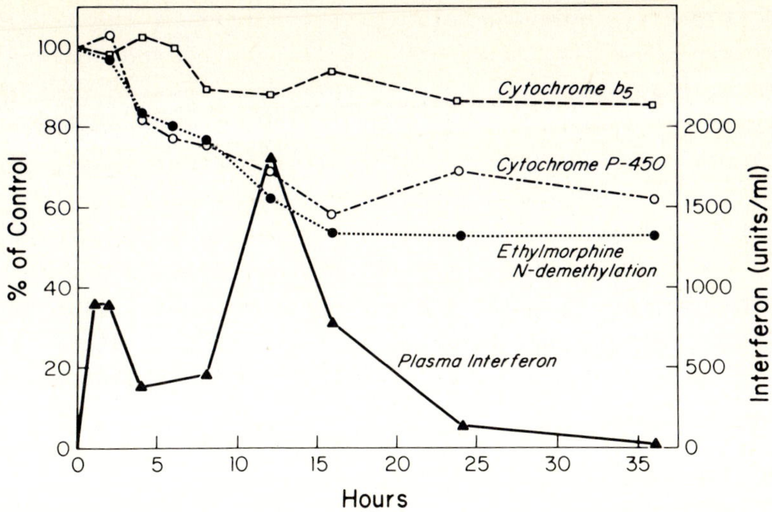

Figure 1 The temporal relationship between the production of interferon and the decrease in hepatic mixed-function oxidase in the mouse following the administration of poly rI.rC (10 mg/kg).

When Newcastle Disease virus was administered to different strains of mice, the lowering of drug biotransformation correlated with the ability of that strain to produce interferon (Singh and Renton, 1981). When C57BL/6J mice which carry an allele (IF-1^h) for high production of interferon were given the virus, large amounts of interferon appeared in the circulation and cytochrome P-450 and drug biotransformation was greatly

Table 2 Correlation of interferon production and loss of cytochrome P-450 in different mouse strains treated with Newcastle Disease Virus.

Strain	Allele	Treatment	Interferon (PRD_{50} units/ml)	Cytochrome P-450
C56BL/6J	1F-1^h	Saline	40	0.63 ± 0.60
C57BC/6J	1F-1^h	NDV	2442 ± 870*	0.40 ± 0.21*
C_3H/HeJ	1F-1^l	Saline	40	0.64 ± 0.42
C_3H/H3J	1F-1^l	NDV	40	0.62 ± 0.38

*Significantly different from corresponding control (n=6).

decreased (Table 2). When C_3H/HeJ mice which carry a low interferon production allele (IF-1^{l}) was used no interferon was produced and no lowering of drug metabolism was observed. It therefore appears that the depression of cytochrome P-450 mediated drug metabolism is decreased as a consequence of the appearance of interferon rather than another aspect of immune function.

Recently we have shown that a highly purified homogeneous human interferon (LeIF-AD) produced from cloned genes depressed the levels of hepatic cytochrome P-450 and related xenobiotic metabolism as shown in Table 3 (Singh, Renton and Stebbing, 1982). Using another cloned human interferon (LeIF-A) several impure preparations of human and mouse

Table 3 The effect of interferon on cytochrome P-450 dependent drug metabolism

Treatment	Cytochrome P-450	Aminopyrine N-demethylase	Anti-viral activity in the mouse
LeIf-AD (40,000 units)	53.0 ± 4.8*	54.5 ± 3.9*	+
LeIF-A (50,000 units)	116.7 ± 4.5	107.1 ± 5.7	-
Human IFN- (50,000 units)	107.0 ± 2.5	103.3 ± 3.0	-
Mouse IFN- (50,000 units)	58.6 ± 2.2*	59.7 ± 2.1*	+
Mouse IFN- (50,000 units)	59.1 ± 4.5*	50.0 ± 4.5*	+
Poly rI.rC (10 mg/kg)	67.7 ± 5.4*	79.7 ± 4.3*	+

Values are the mean ± S.E. of the percentages of control values (n=4).
* Significantly different from control, $p < .05$.

interferon, it appears that only interferons with antiviral activity in the mouse depress cytochrome P-450 in that species. This is the first direct evidence that interferon decreases hepatic drug biotransformation and likely explains the depression of drug elimination which occurs during viral infections or following the administration of interferon inducers.

In man, many reports now exist demonstrating that viral infection can impair the ability of the liver to metabolize and excrete drugs. Of particular note is the reports indicating that influenza infections can alter the elimination of drugs such as theophylline (Renton, 1981). The potential seriousness of such changes is illustrated by Kraemer, Furawaka, Koup, Shapiro, Pierson and Fierman (1982) who reported the occurrence of theophylline toxicity in eleven children during an influenza epidemic in

Seattle in 1980. Each child had no previous problems with their theophylline doses prior to their episode of infection. Also we have shown that the elimination of theophylline in volunteers is impaired following the administration of influenza vaccine (Table 4) (Renton, Gray and Hall, 1981). A dangerous increase in theophylline level was reported by

Table 4 Effect of influenza vaccine on theophylline elimination in human volunteers.

	Control	Influenza Vaccine
Half-Life (hrs)	3.30 ± 0.39	7.30 ± 0.84*
Clearance (ml/kg/hr)	51.6 ± 11.9	25.4 ± 6.3 *
Vd (L/kg)	0.24 ± 0.05	0.25 ± 0.05

*Significantly different from control.
Each value is the mean ± S.E., n=4.

Walker, Schreiber and Middlekamp (1981) in a patient following an influenza vaccination. Kraemer and McClain (1981) have reported that influenza vaccine impaired the metabolism of aminopyrine in 12 volunteers and caused problems in warfarin dosage in a single patient. This effect of influenza vaccine on drug metabolism has been disputed by some reports which found no change in theophylline elimination following vaccination (Fischer, Booth, Mitchell and Kibbe, 1982). It is probable that there are major differences in the types of vaccine used in these studies and that a large study using the various types of vaccine available is required to determine if the effect is confined to only a few types of influenza vaccine.

Although a large number of agents which stimulate host defence mechanisms can impair the cytochrome P-450 drug metabolizing system in the liver, only the production of interferon has been established as a definite mediator of this effect. Although interferon may play a significant role in the decrease in the ability of individuals to eliminate drugs and chemicals during infections, it is unlikely to be the only host defence mechanism which is involved.

REFERENCES

FISHER, R.G., BOOTH, B.H., MITCHELL, D.Q. and KIBBE, A.H. (1982) Influence of trivalent influenza vaccine on serum theophylline levels. Can. Med. Assoc. J. 126, 1312.

KRAEMER, M.J., FURAWAKA, C.T., KOUP, J.R., SHAPIRO, G.G., PIERSON, W.E. and FIERMAN, C.W. (1982) Altered theophylline clearance during an influenza B outbreak. Pediatrics 69, 476.

KRAEMER, P. and McCLAIN, C.J. (1981) Depression of aminopyrine metabolism by influenza vaccination. New Eng. J. Med. 305, 1262.

PETERSON, F.J. and HOLTZMAN, J.L. (1980) Drug Metabolism in the liver. In: Extra hepatic metabolism of drugs and foreign compounds. (ed. Gram, T.E.) Spectrum Publications, N.Y.

RENTON, K.W. (1981) Effects of infection and immune stimulation on theophylline metabolism. Seminars in Perinatology 5, 378.

RENTON, K.W. (1982) Relationships between detoxification enzymes and host defense mechanisms. In: Enzymatic Basis of Detoxification. (eds. Jakoby and Caldwell) Academic Press, N.Y. (in press).

RENTON, K.W., GRAY, J.D. and HALL, R.I. (1981) Decreased elimination of theophylline after influenza vaccination. Can. Med. Assoc. J. 123, 288.

RENTON, K.W. and MANNERING, G.J. (1976) Depression of hepatic cytochrome P-450-dependent monooxygenase systems with administered interferon inducing agents. Biochem. Biophys. Res. Comm. 73, 343.

SINGH, G. and RENTON, K.W. (1981) Interferon-mediated depression of cytochrome P-450-dependent drug biotransformation. Molec. Pharmacol. 20, 681.

SINGH, G., RENTON, K.W. and STEBBING, N. (1982) Homogeneous interferon from E. Coli depresses hepatic cytochrome P-450 and drug biotransformation. Biochem. Biophys. Res. Comm. 106, 1256.

SOYKA, L.F., STEPHENS, C., MacPHERSON, B.R. and FOSTER, R.S. (1979) Role of mononuclear phagocytes in decreased hepatic drug metabolism following administration of Corynebacterium parvum. Int. J. Immunopharmacol. 1, 101.

WALKER, S., SCHREIBER, L. and MIDDLEKAMP, J.N. (1981) Serum theophylline levels after influenza vaccination. Can. Med. Assoc. J. 125, 243.

WILLIAMS, J.F., WINTERS, A.L., LOWITT, S. and SZENTIVANJI, A. (1981) Depression of hepatic mixed function oxidase activity of B. pertussis in splenectomized and athymic nude mice. Immunopharmacol. 3, 101.

APPLICATIONS OF LIPOSOMES IN IMMUNOPOTENTIATION*

P.N. SHEK

Immunology Group, Biosciences Division
Defence and Civil Institute of Environmental Medicine
Department of National Defence, Downsview, Ontario, Canada

LIPOSOMES

Liposomes are membranous vesicles composed predominantly of phospholipids (Bangham, 1972). When dry phospholipids are confronted with an aqueous solution, they undergo a series of rearrangements resulting in the formation of concentric lipid bilayers alternating with aqueous compartments. Upon ultrasonication of these large multilamellar vesicles (MLV, 400-3,500 nm), small unilamellar vesicles (SUV, 20-50 nm) consisting of a single lipid bilayer can be obtained (Huang & Thompson, 1974; Szoka & Papahadjopoulos, 1980). Methods have also been developed for the preparation of large unilamellar vesicles (LUV, 200-1,000 nm) by the fusion of SUV (Papahadjopoulos et al., 1975), by the vaporization of an ether solution of lipid (Deamer & Bangham, 1976), and by the removal of detergent from dissolved lipids (Milsmann, Schweidener & Weder, 1978; Enoch & Strittmatter, 1979). The physical structures of liposomes can be modified in terms of their lipid composition, size, surface charge, and membrane lamellar arrangements. During the process of liposome formation, water-soluble solutes may be entrapped within the aqueous compartments and hydrophobic substances may be incorporated in the lipid bilayers of the vesicle. The attractiveness in the application of liposomes as a carrier system resides in the compatibility of the constituent components with the body system. Being made up of naturally occurring lipid materials, e.g., lecithin and cholesterol, liposomes are biodegradable, relatively non-toxic, and very feebly immunogenic by themselves (Adams et al., 1977; Gregoriadis, 1978; Hart et al., 1981). Liposomes have been used as couriers for a wide variety of materials including enzymes (Gregoriadis & Ryman, 1972; Weissmann et al., 1978), drugs (Rahman et al., 1974; Kimelberg et al., 1976; Fendler & Romero, 1977; Alving et al., 1978; Kaye et al., 1981; Gregoriadis, 1981), protein antigens (Allison & Gregoriadis, 1974; Heath, Edwards

*This is publication number 82-P-22 from the Defence and Civil Institute of Environmental Medicine.

NATO ASI Series, Vol. G2
Immunotoxicology. Edited by P. W. Mullen

& Ryman, 1976; Van Rooijen & Van Nieuwmegen, 1977; Shek & Sabiston, 1982a), and hormones (Patel & Ryman, 1976; Shaw et al., 1976). Among the many potential applications of liposomes in therapeutic and preventive medicine (Ryman & Tyrrell, 1980; Gregoriadis, 1981), the first to be realized may be the use of liposomes as immunopotentiating carriers.

POTENTIATION OF THE ANTIBODY RESPONSE TO LIPOSOME-ASSOCIATED PROTEIN ANTIGENS

The effectiveness of the association of a protein antigen to liposomes in enhancing the anti-protein antibody response was originally described by Allison and Gregoriadis (1974). In contrast to their initial anticipation that the entrapment of an antigen within liposomal vesicles might render it non-immunogenic, it was found that liposome-encapsulated diphtheria toxoid elicited a much higher antibody response against diphtheria than that induced by the free toxoid. The demonstration of the adjuvant effect of liposomes has subsequently been extended to other protein antigens in terms of enhanced circulating antibody titers (Heath et al., 1976; Van Rooijen & Van Nieuwmegen, 1977; Six et al., 1980) and elevated antibody-forming cell response (Shek & Sabiston, 1982a). Unlike other potent immunoadjuvants, e.g., complete Freund's adjuvant, which are unacceptable for human use because of undesirable necrotic reactions at the site of injection, liposome-encapsulated antigens do not induce local granuloma formation (Allison & Gregoriadis, 1976). Another advantage of using liposomes as an immunostimulator is its apparent ineffectiveness in provoking delayed hypersensitivity reactions to the encapsulated antigen (Gregoriadis & Allison, 1974). Furthermore, the lipids used in the synthesis of the commonly used liposomal vesicles are not foreign to the body and no apparent ill effects have been found in injected human subjects (Allison & Gregoriadis, 1976; Richardson et al., 1979; Belchetz et al., 1977). Although liposomal vesicles may prove to be effective and safe vaccine carriers, the critical physicochemical factors of these vesicles in stimulating an optimal response are ill-defined and the cellular mechanisms mediating their immunopotentiating effects have not been established.

Lipid Composition

A variety of lipid constituents has been used in the preparation of liposomes for immunopotentiation. The basic backbone of the liposome is its phospholipid bilayers and the most commonly used phospholipid in liposome preparations is phosphatidylcholine. Some examples of phosphatidylcholine-containing liposomes that have been found effective in immunopotentiation are

TABLE I

LIPID COMPOSITION OF LIPOSOMES EFFECTIVE IN POTENTIATING THE ANTIBODY RESPONSE TO SOME PROTEIN ANTIGENS

Protein Antigens	Lipid composition	References
Diphtheria toxoid	7PC:2CSL:1DCP 7PC:2CSL:1PA	Allison & Gregoriadis, 1974 Allison & Gregoriadis, 1976
Bovine serum albumin	9PC:1DCP 7PC:2CSL:1PA	Heath *et al.*, 1976 Shek & Sabiston, 1982a
Human serum albumin	7PC:2CSL:1PA	Van Rooijen & Van Nieuwmegen, 1977
Bovine gamma globulin	7PC:2CSL:1PA	Van Rooijen & Van Nieuwmegen, 1980
Hepatitis B surface antigen	7PC:2CSL:1DCP	Gregoriadis & Manesis, 1980
Adenovirus protein antigen	10DPPC:7.5CSL:1PA	Six *et al.*, 1980
Gross-virus cell surface antigen	7PC:2CSL:1DCP	Gerlier *et al.*, 1980

PC, phosphatidylcholine; DPPC, dipalmitoyl phosphatidylcholine; CSL, cholesterol; DCP, dicetyl phosphate; PA, phosphatidic acid.

listed in Table I. In most studies, the molar ratio of the lipids used is empirically determined. Nevertheless, liposomes of varied lipid composition and surface charge are capable of enhancing the antibody response to a number of protein antigens. The incorporation of cholesterol in the liposomal membrane enhances the structural integrity of the lipid bilayer (Finkelstein & Weissmann, 1979) and a high cholesterol/phospholipid ratio reduces the permeability of the vesicle (Papahadjopoulos *et al.*, 1972). Although a relatively high cholesterol content was reported to reduce the antibody response to the entrapped antigen (Heath *et al.*, 1976), the critical role of cholesterol in supporting the adjuvanticity of liposomes has not been analyzed. It has been reported that the immunogenicity of hapten-substituted liposomes is related to the lipid composition and the phase-transition temperatures of the phospholipids used (Yasuda *et al.*, 1977; Van Houte *et al.*, 1981); however, similar studies have not been conducted for liposome-associated protein antigens. It is of interest to note that haptenated liposomes prepared from glycerophospholipid are much less efficient than those prepared from sphingophospholipid in potentiating the hapten-specific antibody response (Yasuda *et al.*, 1977). In contrast, phosphatidylcholine liposomes are more potent than sphingomyelin liposomes in promoting antibody formation to liposome-associated protein antigens (Heath *et al.*, 1976).

The introduction of surface charge to liposomal vesicles may result in different potentiating effects. Thus, positively-charged liposomes were found ineffective in promoting the anti-diphtheria antibody response (Allison & Gregoriadis, 1974) but were proficient in enhancing the antibody response to serum albumin (Heath et al., 1976). The incorporation of a charged lipid results in the bilayers repelling one another and this increases the entrapped aqueous space (Bangham et al., 1967). The extent to which charged vesicles interact electrostatically with proteins varies, depending on the isoelectric point of the protein involved. Thus, surface charge characteristics not only affect the extent of protein entrapment but also influence the non-covalent interactions of the lipid bilayers with the protein antigen. The nature of association between the vesicle and the antigen may influence the resulting antigenicity of the liposome-associated protein.

MLV versus LUV

Most studies conducted to investigate the adjuvant effect of liposomes invariably used MLV as antigen carriers. This may stem from their ease of preparation and their sufficient effectiveness in potentiating the immunogenicity of the antigen being examined. In order to determine whether the lamellar structure of liposomal carriers may influence the magnitude of the provoked antibody response, MLV and LUV of approximately the same size range were used to compare their efficacy in promoting the response to their entrapped antigens. It can be seen from Table II that LUV is much more effective than MLV in potentiating the plaque-forming cell (PFC) response to the entrapped bovine serum albumin (BSA) in mice. The reason for this difference is not known. However, LUV has been shown to have a larger captured volume than MLV resulting in a higher efficiency of encapsulation (Papahadjopoulos et al., 1980). Furthermore, the uptake of entrapped antigen by phagocytic cells is proportional to the captured volume of the vesicle (Poste et al, 1980). Thus, in all likelihood, the entrapped antigen of LUV should be more readily available to the interacting cell, e.g., a macrophage, since the vesicle is enclosed by only a single lipid bilayer. Alternatively, the difference in immunoenhancing capacity between MLV and LUV may be related to different patterns of homing to the target lymphoid organ.

TABLE II

ANTI-BSA PFC RESPONSE ELICITED BY MLV- AND LUV-ASSOCIATED BSA IN A/J MICE

Antigen[a]	Number of Mice	BSA-specific IgG PFC/spleen[b]	p[c]
MLV-BSA	8	59,200 ± 7,600	
LUV-BSA	8	139,000 ± 15,000	< 0.0005

[a] BSA was entrapped in MLV (330 ± 70 nm) or LUV (240 ± 50 nm) composed of dimyristoyl phosphatidylcholine, cholesterol and dicetyl phosphate in a molar ratio of 7:2:1. Mice were given 2 identical intraperitoneal injections, 3 weeks apart, of each antigen preparation containing 30 μg of BSA protein.

[b] Splenic BSA-specific PFC response was assayed 4 days after the second injection of antigen.

[c] p value (Student's t-test) comparing the PFC response of the two groups.

Site of Association

One crucial parameter which determines the effectiveness of liposomes in potentiating the antibody response to an antigen is the physical association between the two entities. Although liposome-associated BSA consistently elicited an enhanced anti-BSA antibody response, the separate but simultaneous injection of liposomes and the free BSA (fBSA) failed to elicit an appreciable response (Fig. 1). Thus, a direct physical association of the antigen with the liposomal vesicle is imperative for successful immunopotentiation to occur. Although physical linkage between the antigen and the liposome is essential, opposite views have been expressed regarding the importance of the actual site of association. Using different liposome-antigen systems, suggestions were put forward favouring either internal entrapment (Six et al., 1980) or surface adsorption of the antigen (Van Rooijen & Van Nieuwmegen, 1980) as being essential in liposome-mediated enhancement. In order to investigate this apparent discrepancy, the relative immunogenicity of a protein antigen associated with liposomes on the surface or entrapped internally was compared under one experimental system. Different preparations of the appropriate liposome-associated BSA antigens used are shown in Fig. 2. It was found that animals immunized with liposomes, containing both entrapped and surface-adsorbed BSA, $(LSM\text{-}BSA)_{e+a}$, gave a BSA-specific PFC response comparable to that elicited by animals immunized with trypsinized $(LSM\text{-}BSA)_{e+a}$ which contained mainly entrapped BSA (Fig. 3). In contrast, the PFC response elicited by animals immunized with liposomes containing only BSA adsorbed on the membrane surface, $(LSM\text{-}BSA)_a$, was significantly less than that of

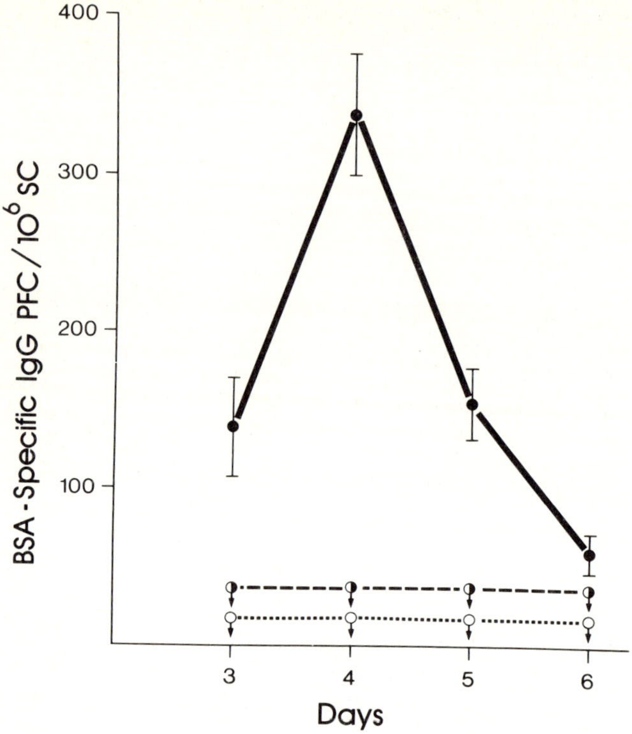

Figure 1. Potentiation of the BSA-specific PFC response by LSM-BSA. A/J mice were given two intraperitoneal injections of 50 μg of either LSM-BSA (●), fBSA (○), or fBSA together with empty LSM (◑), 2 weeks apart. Spleen cells of the immunized animals were harvested for the PFC assay 3-6 days after the second injection of antigen. Each point represents the mean response ± SEM of seven to ten animals. The inverted arrow indicates a mean response of less than 10 PFC per 10^6 spleen cells. (From Shek & Sabiston, 1982a).

the above two groups. Finally, animals injected with trypsinized $(LSM\text{-}BSA)_a$ only elicited a marginally detectable PFC response. These results demonstrate that liposomes are effective in potentiating the antibody response to the associated protein antigen irrespective of the site of association, although the entrapped antigen appears to be more immunogenic.

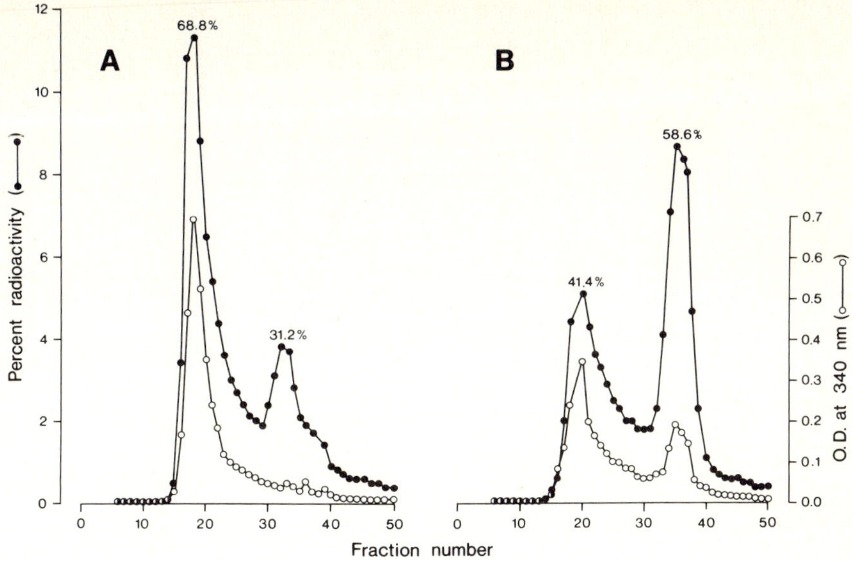

Figure 2a. Sepharose-4B chromatography of A: $(LSM\text{-}BSA)_{e+a}$ and B: trypsinized $(LSM\text{-}BSA)_{e+a}$. A dried lipid film, composed of phosphatidylcholine, cholesterol, and phosphatidic acid in a molar ratio of 7:2:1, was resuspended in a protein solution containing unlabelled BSA (12 mg/ml) and ^{125}I-labelled BSA (14.2 Ci/mmol). After an incubation period of 2 hr at room temperature, the liposomal suspension was sonicated (100 watts, 30 sec) and most of the protein molecules not associated with the liposome were removed by centrifugation at 100,000 g for 30 min. The resulting liposomal pellet which contained entrapped and surface adsorbed BSA molecules, $(LSM\text{-}BSA)_{e+a}$, was resuspended and divided into two equal aliquots. One aliquot was passed through a Sepharose-4B column (1.5 x 30 cm) equilibrated with 0.15M phosphate-buffered saline, pH 7.2 (panel A) and the other aliquot was treated with trypsin before its passage through the same column (panel B). Fractions of 2 ml were collected and protein recovery in each fraction was expressed as a percentage of the recovered radioactivity. The percentage figure indicated at the top of each peak represents the summation of the total radioactivity of the fractions of that peak.

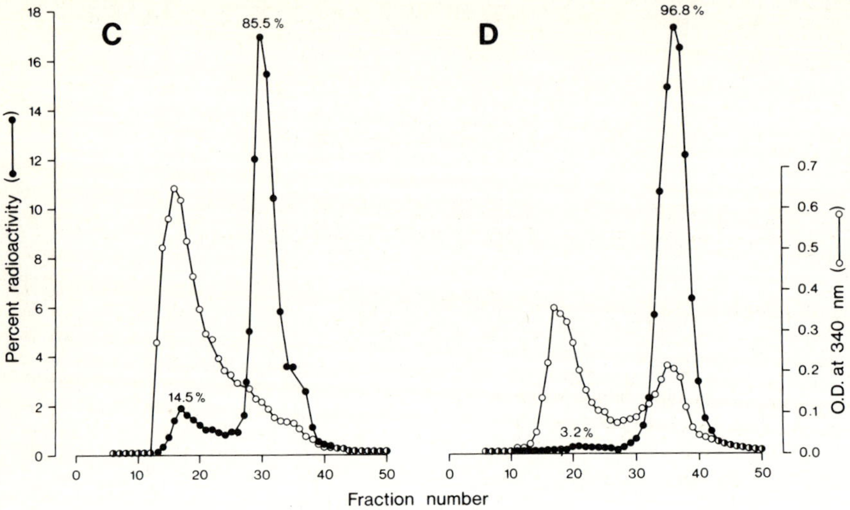

Figure 2b. Sepharose-4B chromatography of C: $(LSM\text{-}BSA)_a$, and D: trypsinized $(LSM\text{-}BSA)_a$. Preformed empty liposomes, composed of phosphatidylcholine, cholesterol, and phosphatidic acid in a molar ratio of 7:2:1, were mixed with a protein solution containing unlabelled BSA (12 mg/ml) and ^{125}I-labelled BSA (14.2 Ci/mmol). After an incubation period of 2 hr at room temperature, the liposomal suspension was sonicated (100 watts, 30 sec) and most of the protein molecules not associated with the liposomes were removed by centrifugation at 100,000 g for 30 min. The resulting liposomal pellet which contained surface-adsorbed BSA molecules, $(LSM\text{-}BSA)_a$, was resuspended and divided into two equal aliquots. One aliquot was passed through a Sepharose-4B column (1.5 x 30 cm) equilibrated with 0.15M phosphate-buffered saline, pH 7.2 (panel C) and the other aliquot was treated with trypsin before its passage through the same column (panel D). Fractions were collected and monitored as described in Fig. 2a (From Shek & Sabiston, 1982b).

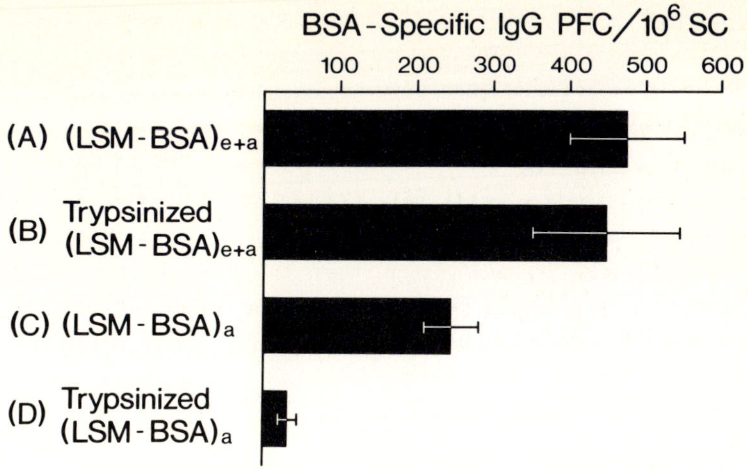

Figure 3. BSA-specific PFC response to immunizations with 4 preparations of liposome-associated BSA antigen. Different groups of A/J mice were given two intraperitoneal injections, 0.5 mg per injection, of one of the LSM-BSA preparations, 3 weeks apart. Each LSM-BSA preparation was obtained from the pooled fractions of the excluded peak of the corresponding chromatographic run shown in Fig. 2. Immunized animals were killed 4 days after the second injection of antigen and their spleen cells were harvested for the PFC assay. Comparison of the mean PFC response by Student's t-test between groups: A and B (not significant); A and C ($p < 0.01$); C and D ($p < 0.001$) (From Shek & Sabiston, 1982b).

Route of Administration

The administration of liposome-associated antigens via the intraperitoneal, subcutaneous, intramuscular, and intravenous routes has been found to be effective in enhancing the antibody response. Although the intravenous route was considered to be a poor way of immunizing mice with liposome-entrapped antigen (Tyrrell et al., 1976), consistent immunoenhancement was obtained in rabbits via this route (Van Rooijen & Van Nieuwmegen, 1977). Immunization of mice by subcutaneous injections with liposome-associated albumin elicited a higher antibody titer than via the intravenous route (Heath et al., 1976), but the reverse appears to be true if the entrapped antigen is diphtheria toxoid (Allison & Gregoriadis, 1976). Most likely, the route of antigen administration is not the only parameter which determines the magnitude of immunoenhancement. Other factors, such as the physicochemical properties of the liposomal carrier, the biochemical nature of the protein antigen used, the mode of liposome-antigen association, and the dose of antigen employed, may also contribute to modulating the immunostimulatory effect.

T-Cell Dependency

The antibody response to most protein antigens, e.g., BSA, requires the participation of thymus-derived (T) cells (Taylor, 1969; Allison & Davis, 1971). Since it has been reported that the hapten-specific PFC response to haptenated liposomes does not require T-cell help (Yasuda et al., 1979; Van Houte et al., 1979), the question arises whether liposome-encapsulated protein antigens can become T-independent. It was found that the immunization of animals with liposome-associated BSA failed to induce either a primary (Table III) or secondary (Shek & Sabiston, 1982a) anti-BSA PFC response in congenitally athymic nude

TABLE III

COMPARISON OF ANTIGEN-SPECIFIC PRIMARY PFC RESPONSE TO LSM-BSA AND TKS AMONG NORMAL BALB/c MICE, HOMOZYGOUS ATHYMIC NUDE (Nu/Nu) MICE, AND HETEROZYGOUS (Nu/+) LITTERMATES

Strain[a]	Antigen	PFC Response	p[f]
		BSA-specific PFC/spleen[c]	
BALB/c (+/+)	LSM-BSA[b]	5,570 ± 640	
BALB/c (Nu/+)	LSM-BSA	4,930 ± 490	n.s.
BALB/c (Nu/Nu)	LSM-BSA	30 ± 10	$<$ 0.0001
		TNP-specific PFC/spleen[e]	
BALB/c (+/+)	TKS[d]	11,380 ± 590	
BALB/c (Nu/+)	TKS	13,500 ± 650	n.s.
BALB/c (Nu/Nu)	TKS	11,150 ± 920	n.s.

[a] 5 animals in each group.

[b] 50 μg LSM-BSA injected intraperitoneally.

[c] BSA-specific indirect PFC response was assayed 6 days after immunization.

[d] 100 μg TNP-KLH-Sepharose (2,4,6-trinitrophenylated keyhole-limpet-hemocyanin-conjugated Sepharose, a T-cell independent antigen) injected intraperitoneally.

[e] TNP-specific direct PFC was assayed 8 days after immunization.

[f] p value (Student's t-test) in comparison to the corresponding PFC response of normal BALB/c (+/+) animals.

(Nu/Nu) mice. This provides direct evidence demonstrating the obligatory role of T cells in mediating the immunostimulatory effect of liposomes for encapsulated protein antigens. It is possible that entrapped protein antigens are not directly accessible to B cells; whereas, the substitution of haptenic molecules, especially at high epitope densities, on the liposome surface, may facilitate the direct activation of B cells. Another line of observation which implicates thymic involvement in immunopotentiation, mediated by liposome-associated protein antigen, is the capacity of encapsulated antigen to generate a strong immunological memory. It is evident from Fig. 4 that mice previously primed with liposome-associated BSA elicited an intensive secondary PFC response, even when challenged with the weakly immunogenic free BSA. The amplification of an anamnestic IgG response requires the modulation of long-lived recirculating memory T cells (Miller, 1973). Thus, our data appear to suggest that liposome-encapsulated protein antigen is proficient in provoking a thymic-dependent memory.

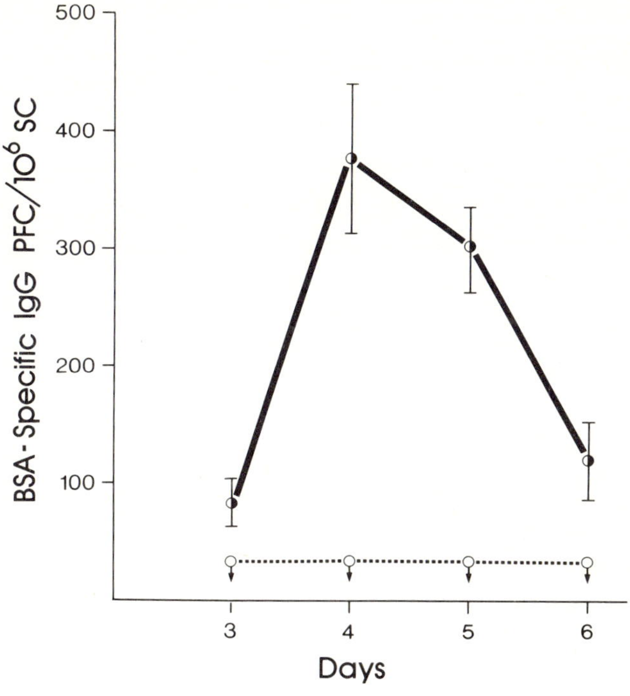

Figure 4. Effectiveness of LSM-BSA in priming animals for a secondary antibody response. A/J mice were divided into two groups and each group was injected intraperitoneally with 50 μg of either LSM-BSA (◑), or free BSA (○). After a resting period of 5 weeks, all animals were challenged with 50 μg of free BSA. The spleen cells of the immunized animals were harvested for the PFC assay 3-6 days after antigenic challenge. Each point represents the mean response ± SEM of five to six animals. The inverted arrow indicates a mean response of less than 10 PFC per 10^6 spleen cells (From Shek & Sabiston, 1982a).

Role of Macrophages

In view of the fact that T cells are required in promoting the antibody response to liposome-encapsulated protein antigens, the involvement of an accessory cell, e.g., macrophage, in antigen processing is very likely. In order to determine whether macrophage participation is essential, the effect of the depletion of macrophages on the antibody response to liposome-entrapped proteins was studied. The abrogation of macrophage function was achieved by the *in vivo* administration of carrageenan, a sulfated polygalactose. Carrageenan is cytotoxic for phagocytic cells, but exerts no harmful effect on lymphocytes (Cantanzaro *et al.*, 1971; Ishizaka *et al.*, 1977; Thomson *et al.*, 1979). It is evident from Fig. 5 that the injection of mice with carrageenan suppressed their PFC response to sheep red blood cells (SRBC), a macrophage-dependent T-cell antigen (Mitchell & Miller, 1968; Gorcynski *et al.*, 1971) but had no effect on the response to *E. coli* lipopolysaccharide, a macrophage-independent B-cell antigen (Wong & Herscowitz, 1979). The pretreatment of mice with carrageenan suppressed their PFC response to liposome-entrapped BSA (Table IV) and abolished their circulating anti-BSA antibody titers (Fig. 6). Our results support the view that macrophages play an obligatory role in mediating the antibody response to liposome-associated protein antigens. *In vitro* studies on the immunogenicity of haptenated liposomes also demonstrate the requirement of macrophages for successful induction of a hapten-specific PFC response, but the macrophage requirement can be replaced by the addition of 2-mercaptoethanol (Yasuda *et al.*, 1979) or of a soluble factor released by Concanavalin A-stimulated spleen cells (Humphries, 1981).

Vaccine Carrier

An ideal vaccine carrier is one which is capable of potentiating the immunogenicity of purified vaccine subunits or specific antigenic determinants, without provoking undesirable local and systemic allergic reactions. The carrier itself should be harmless, non-foreign to the body, and easily metabolized. Being composed of naturally-occurring lipids, appropriately prepared liposomes possess most, if not all, of these desirable features. Phosphatidylcholine, the most commonly used phospholipid for liposome preparations, is practically non-immunogenic by itself (Gregoriadis, 1978; Scherphof *et al.*, 1981). The modification of phosphatidylcholine liposomes by the incorporation, in the lipid bilayers, of other adjuvant substances, e.g., lipid A of bacterial lipopolysaccharide, however, can induce the formation of anti-liposome antibodies (Schuster *et al.*, 1979). Thus, the lipid composition of a vaccine carrier should be chosen to

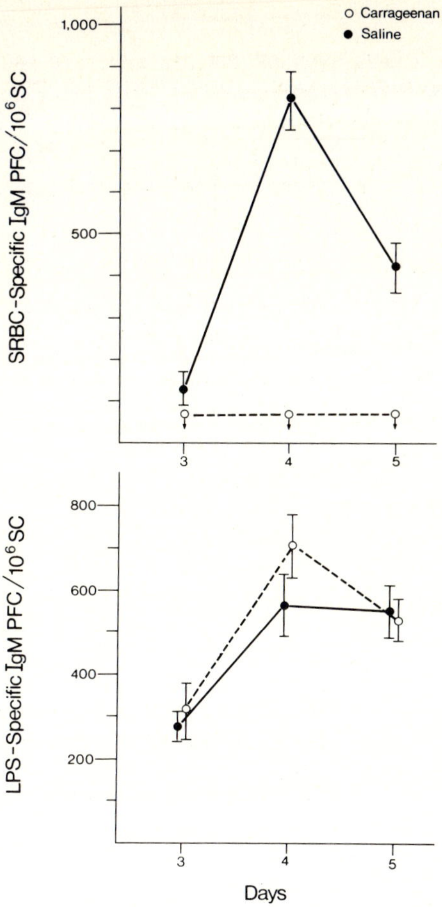

Figure 5. Effect of carrageenan on the PFC response to SRBC and LPS *in vivo*. Different groups of A/J mice were given two intraperitoneal injections of carrageenan, 0.5 mg per injection, 5 and 2 days before their immunizations with either 5 x 10^8 SRBC, a macrophage-dependent antigen, or 10 μg of *E. coli* LPS, a macrophage-independent antigen. Animals in each control group were similarly immunized but the pretreatment with carrageenan was replaced by the injection of saline. The SRBC-specific (upper panel) and LPS-specific (lower panel) PFC response of the injected animals was assayed 3 to 5 days after antigen challenge. Each point represents the mean PFC response ± SEM of 6 to 8 animals (From Shek & Lukovich, 1982).

TABLE IV

IN VIVO SUPPRESSION OF THE BSA-SPECIFIC PFC RESPONSE BY THE ADMINISTRATION OF CARRAGEENAN IN A/J MICE

Treatment[a]		Antigen	BSA-specific indirect PFC/spleen		p[d]
Day -5	Day -2	Day 0	Day 6		
Saline	Saline	LSM-BSA[b]	6,040 ± 360	(6)[c]	
Carrageenan	carrageenan	LSM-BSA	84 ± 16	(6)	<0.0001

[a] Animals were injected intraperitoneally with either saline or 0.5 mg of carrageenan each time on day -5 and day -2 before immunization.

[b] Immunized intraperitoneally with 50 μg LSM-BSA.

[c] Number of animals in each group.

[d] p value (Student's t-test) comparing the PFC response of the two groups.

eliminate or to minimize the induction of antibody formation against the membrane components.

So far, all studies investigating the efficacy of liposomes as an immunopotentiating carrier have been conducted by parenteral immunizations. The potential in the application of liposomal vesicles as a vaccine carrier for oral immunization has not been explored. In regard to this approach, it has been reported that oral administration of liposome-encapsulated biological compounds such as insulin (Patel & Ryman, 1976) and factor VIII (Hemker et al., 1980) resulted in the absorption, though in limited amounts, of the active compound from the gastrointestinal tract into the circulation. The use of liposomes as a vaccine carrier for oral immunization will most likely promote IgA immunity. However, if sufficient entrapped antigenic materials find their way to non-gut-associated lymphoid organs, e.g., the spleen, via the lymphatics and the blood stream, the formation of antibodies of IgM and IgG classes may also be enhanced. The development of a suitable liposomal vaccine carrier for oral immunization undoubtedly requires the engineering of a vesicle with appropriate physicochemical characteristics which favour immunopotentiation via the gastrointestinal tract.

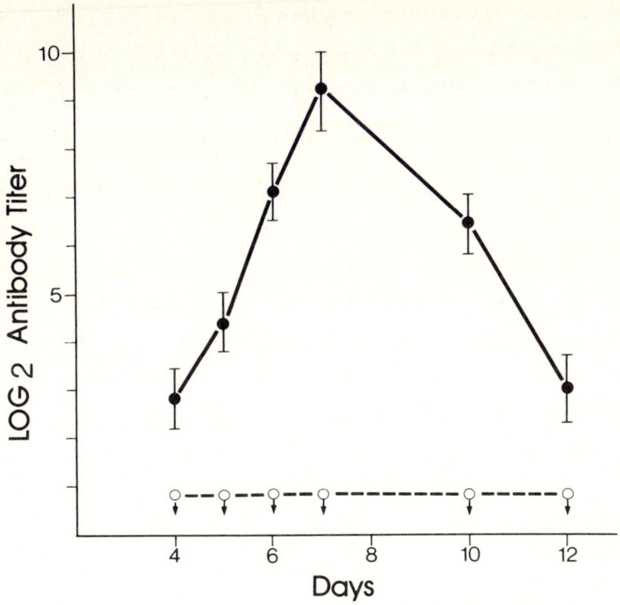

Figure 6. Suppression of circulating anti-BSA antibody titers by the administration of carrageenan *in vivo*. A/J mice in the experimental group (○) were injected intraperitoneally twice with carrageenan, 0.5 mg per injection, 5 and 2 days before their immunizations with 50 μg of LSM-BSA. Animals in the control group (●) were similarly immunized except the pretreatment was replaced with saline. The immunized animals were bled at different time intervals after immunization. Each point represents the mean serum anti-BSA hemagglutinating antibody titers of 6 animals. The inverted arrow indicates no detectable antibody titer.

POTENTIATION OF CELL-MEDIATED IMMUNITY

In addition to their ability to enhance antibody formation, liposomes are also effective in promoting cell-mediated immunity. Different types of cellular responses induced by liposome-associated macromolecules have been studied.

Proliferative Response

The proliferative response of cultured lymphocytes challenged with antigen is considered an *in vitro* correlate of cell-mediated immunity (Bloom, 1971). The extent of cellular multiplication can be determined by measuring the incorporation of tritiated thymidine into DNA of the dividing cells. In an attempt to evaluate the efficacy of liposome-associated antigen in eliciting a primarily T-cell proliferative response, rabbits were immunized in one foot pad with liposome-encapsulated BSA and cells from the draining popliteal lymph node were subsequently cultured in the presence of the antigen. It is evident that lymph node cells, primed with liposome-entrapped BSA, elicited a significantly higher proliferative response than cells obtained from the control lymph node primed with free BSA (Fig. 7). It has been demonstrated that liposomes injected via the foot pad are localized predominantly in the regional lymph nodes (Ryman et al., 1978). This selective localization of the liposome-entrapped antigen may partly explain its apparently better efficacy in provoking a higher response. In contrast, the free antigen may channel through the lymph node more rapidly resulting in less antigen retention by the regional lymphoid cells. Since the T-cell proliferative response is facilitated by the participation of macrophages (Suzuki & Tomasi Jr, 1980), liposome-encapsulated antigen, being in particulate form, is more likely to enhance the uptake by phagocytic cells which in turn triggers an elevated T-cell response.

Induction of Cytotoxic T Lymphocytes

Liposomes have been shown to be effective carriers of major histocompatibility complex (MHC) antigens in inducing the formation of MHC-restricted cytotoxic T lymphocytes (CTL) in murine (Finberg et al., 1978) and human (Engelhard et al., 1978; Burakoff et al., 1980) systems. Previous attempts to investigate the molecular interactions in eliciting the CTL response were hampered by the necessity of using intact cells or cell membranes containing the stimulating antigens. Recent advances in liposome technology enable the incorporation of highly purified recognition molecules, e.g., MHC antigens, cell surface membrane components, and viral antigens in phospholipid vesicles that are capable of triggering the T-cell effector function. The presence of both viral and MHC antigens in liposomes is necessary for the successful stimulation of secondary CTL against specific viral targets (Finberg et al., 1978; Hale et al., 1980). The generation of the CTL response by liposome-incorporated MHC antigen requires the active participation of macrophages (Weinberger et al., 1980). Macrophages are involved in processing the liposome-associated antigen and in activating helper T cells which promote the CTL response (Weinberger et al., 1981).

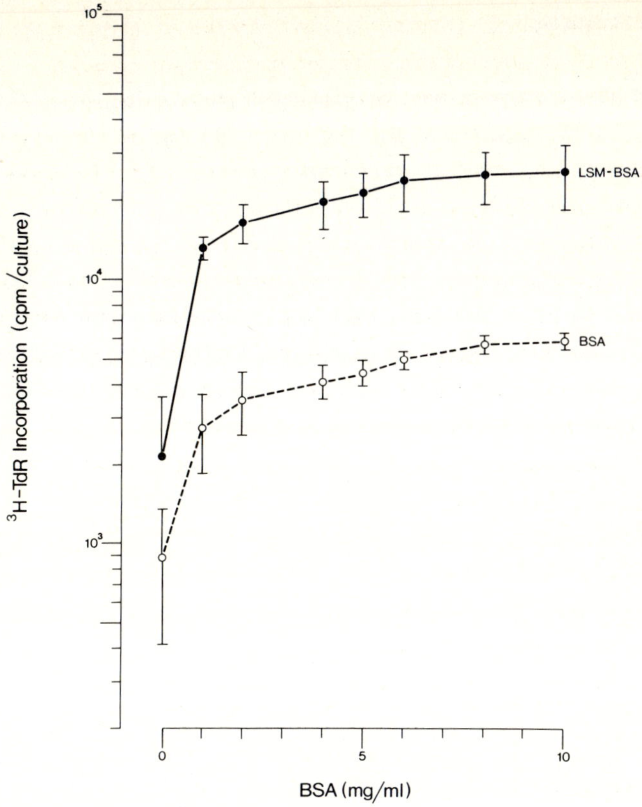

Figure 7. Potentiation of the proliferative response by liposome-associated BSA. Rabbits were immunized with 50 μg of LSM-BSA in one hind foot-pad, and 50 μg of free BSA in the other. Cells from each draining popliteal lymph node were assayed for their *in vitro* BSA-specific proliferative response 3 weeks after immunization. The total culture period was 72 hr and ^{3}H-TdR was added 18 hr before cell harvest. Each point represents the mean cpm ± SEM of 3 animals.

Macrophage Activation

Cell-mediated immunity may be expressed either by the direct action of the effector cell on the target, e.g., the lytic action on the viral target by CTL, or by the release of biologically-active soluble factors, called lymphokines, from activated lymphocytes which are predominantly T cells. One of the many lymphokines obtainable from lymphocytes stimulated by antigens or mitogens is the macrophage activating factor (MAF). Macrophages stimulated by the appropriate lymphokine are more active than resting macrophages in performing phagocytic functions. It is known that MAF-activated macrophages selectively destroy neoplastic, but not normal, cells (Fidler, 1978). The tumoricidal activity of macrophages activated by liposome-encapsulated MAF was much enhanced compared with the free factor (Poste et al., 1980). Using a tumor model in mice, it has been demonstrated that tumor metastasis can be eradicated by activating the tumoricidal functions of macrophages with liposome-encapsulated lymphokines (Fidler et al., 1980). These studies raise hope for the clinical application of liposome-encapsulated lymphokines in the treatment of metastatic tumors.

CONCLUDING REMARKS

In the preceding sections, the efficacy of liposomes in potentiating the humoral and cell-mediated immune response has been presented. It is clear that the versatility of phospholipid vesicles resides in the ease of altering their physicochemical characteristics for specific needs. The lipid composition and physical structure of a liposomal carrier can be adjusted to minimize its intrinsic immunogenicity yet retains its maximal adjuvant effect. Although the cell types involved in interacting with liposome-associated antigens and lymphokines are being identified, the basic mechanisms at the cellular and molecular levels mediating the potentiated response remain ill-defined. The elucidation of the relationship between the nature of liposome/antigen interactions and the potentiated immune response will facilitate a better design of vaccine carriers for human use. In view of the success, though limited, in using liposomal carriers for the delivery of labile substances via the gastrointestinal tract, the development of a suitable lipid vesicle for the delivery of oral vaccines may be on the horizon. Finally, the application of liposomal carriers for the delivery of other biological macromolecules must take into consideration the impact of potential immunological complications.

ACKNOWLEDGEMENTS

The author wishes to thank Ms. D. Kerrigan for her excellent technical assistance and Ms. D. Gardham for her meticulous effort in the preparation of this manuscript.

REFERENCES

ADAMS D.H., JOYCE G., RICHARDSON V.J., RYMAN B.E. & WISNIEWSKI H.M. (1977) Liposome toxicity in the mouse nervous system. J. Neurol. Sci. 31, 173.

ALLISON A.C. & DAVIES A.J.S. (1971) Requirement of thymus-dependent lymphocytes for potentiation by adjuvants of antibody formation. Nature (Lond.) 233, 330.

ALLISON A.C. & GREGORIADIS G. (1974) Liposomes as immunological adjuvants. Nature (Lond.) 252, 252.

ALLISON A.C. & GREGORIADIS G. (1976) Liposomes as immunological adjuvants. In: Recent Results in Cancer Research, p. 58. (Ed. by G. Mathe, I. Florentin and M.C. Simmler). Springer-Verlag, Heidelberg.

ALVING C.R., STECK E.A., CHAPMAN JR W.L., WAITS V.B., HENDRICKS L.D., SWARTZ JR G.M. & HANSON W.L. (1978) Therapy of leishmaniasis: superior efficacies of liposome encapsulated drugs. Proc. Natl. Acad. Sci., USA, 75, 2959.

BANGHAM A.D. (1972) Lipid bilayers and biomembranes. Annu. Rev. Biochem. 41, 753.

BANGHAM A.D., DE GIER J. & GREVILLE G.D. (1967) Osmotic properties and water permeability of phospholipid liquid crystals. Chem. Phys. Lipids 1, 225.

BELCHETZ P.E., BRAIDMAN I.P., CRAWLEY J.C.E. & GREGORIADIS G. (1977) Treatment of Gaucher's disease with liposome-entrapped glucocerebroside: beta-glucosidase. Lancet 1, 116.

BLOOM, R.R. (1971) In vitro approaches to the mechanism of cell-mediated immune reactions. Adv. Immunol. 13, 101.

BURAKOFF S.J., ENGELHARD V.H., KAUFMAN J. & STROMINGER J.L. (1980) Induction of secondary cytotoxic T lymphocytes by liposomes containing HLA-DR antigens. Nature 283, 495.

CATANZARO P.J., SCHWARTZ H.J. & GRAHAM R.C. (1971) Spectrum and possible mechanism of carrageenan cytotoxicity. Am. J. Pathol. 64, 387.

DEAMER D. & BANGHAM A.D. (1976) Large volume liposomes by an ether vaporization method. Biochim. Biophys. Acta 443, 629.

ENGELHARD V.H., STROMINGER J.L., MESCHER M. & BURAKOFF S. (1978) Induction of secondary cytotoxic T lymphocytes by purified HLA-A and HLA-B antigens reconstituted into phospholipid vesicles. Proc. Natl. Acad. Sci., USA 75, 5688.

ENOCH H.G. & STRITTMATTER P. (1979) Formation and properties of 1,000 A diameter single bilayer phospholipid vesicles. Proc. Natl. Acad. Sci., USA 76, 145.

FENDLER J.H. & ROMERO A. (1977) Liposomes as drug carriers. Life Sci. 20, 1109.

FIDLER I.J. (1978) Recognition and destruction of target cells by tumoricidal macrophages. Isr. J. Med. Sci. 14, 177.

FIDLER I.J., HART I.R., RAZ A., FOGLER W.E., KIRSH R. & POSTE G. (1980) Activation of tumoricidal properties in macrophages by liposome-encapsulated lymphokines: in vivo studies. In: Liposomes and Immunobiology, p. 109. (Ed. by B.H. Tom and H.R. Six). Elsevier/North Holland, New York.

FINBERG R., MESCHER M. & BURAKOFF S.J. (1978) The induction of virus specific cytotoxic T lymphocytes with solubilized viral and membrane proteins. J. Exp. Med. 148, 1620.

FINKELSTEIN M. & WEISSMANN G. (1979) Enzyme replacement via liposomes. Variations in lipid composition determine liposomal integrity in biological fluids. Biochim. Biophys. Acta 587, 202.

GERLIER D., SAKAI F. & DORE J.F. (1980) Induction of antibody response to liposome-associated Gross-virus cell-surface antigen (GCSAa). Br. J. Cancer 41, 236.

GORCYNSKI R.M., MILLER R.G. & PHILLIPS R.A. (1971) In vivo requirement for a radiation-resistant cell in the immune response to sheep erythrocytes. J. Exp. Med. 134, 1201.

GREGORIADIS G. (1978) Liposomes in therapeutic and preventive medicine: The development of the drug-carrier concept. Ann. N.Y. Acad. Sci. 308, 343.

GREGORIADIS G. (1981) Targeting of drugs: Implications in medicine. Lancet 2, 241.

GREGORIADIS G. & ALLISON A.C. (1974) Entrapment of proteins in liposomes prevents allergic reactions in pre-immunized mice. FEBS Lett. 45, 71.

GREGORIADIS G. & MANESIS E.K. (1980) Liposomes as immunological adjuvants for hepatitis B surface antigens. In: Liposomes and Immunobiology, p. 271. (Ed. by B.H. Tom and H.R. Six). Elsevier/North Holland, New York.

GREGORIADIS G. & RYMAN B.E. (1972) Fate of protein-containing liposomes injected into rats. An approach to the treatment of storage diseases. Eur. J. Biochem. 24, 485.

HALE A.H., RUEBUSH M.J. & HARRIS D.T. (1980) Study of the minimal molecular and cellular requirement for elicitation of anti-vesicular stomatitis virus cytotoxic T lymphocytes using purified viral and cellular antigens incorporated into phospholipid vesicles. In: Liposomes and Immunobiology, p. 211. (Ed. by B.H. Tom and H.R. Six). Elsevier/North Holland, New York.

HART I.R., FOGLER W.E., POSTE G. & FIDLER I.J. (1981) Toxicity studies of liposome-encapsulated immunomodulators administered intravenously to dogs and mice. Cancer Immunol. Immunother. 10, 157.

HEATH T.D., EDWARDS D.C. & RYMAN B.E. (1976) The adjuvant properties of liposomes. Biochem. Soc. Trans. 4, 129.

HEMKER H.C., HERMENS W.T.H., MULLER A.D. & ZWAAL R.F.A. (1980) Oral treatment of haemophilia A by gastrointestinal absorption of factor VIII entrapped in liposomes. Lancet 1, 70.

HUANG C. & THOMPSON T.E. (1974) Preparation of homogeneous single walled phosphatidylcholine vesicles. Methods Enzymol. 32, 485.

HUMPHRIES G.M.K. (1981) Evidence for direct control of an in vitro plaque-forming cell response by quantitative properties of intact, fluid, haptenated liposomes: A potential model system for antigen presentation by macrophages. J. Immunol. 126, 688.

ISHIZAKA S., OTANI S. & MORISAWA S. (1977) Effects of carrageenan on immune reponses. I. Studies on the macrophage dependency of various antigens after treatment with carrageenan. J. Immunol. 118, 1213.

KAYE S.B., BODEN J.A. & RYMAN B.E. (1981) The effect of liposome entrapment of actinomycin D and methotrexate on the in vivo treatment of sensitive and resistant solid murine tumours. Eur. J. Cancer 17, 279.

KIMELBERG H.K., TRACY T.F., BIDDLECOME S.M. & BOURKE R.S. (1976) The effect of entrapment in liposomes on the in vivo distribution of [^{3}H]methotrexate in a primate. Cancer Res. 36, 2949.

MILLER J.F.A.P. (1973) Immunological memory. Contemp. Top. Immunobiol. 2, 151.

MILSMANN M.H.W., SCHWEIDENER R.A. & WEDER H.G. (1978) The preparation of large single bilayer liposomes by a fast and controlled dialysis. Biochim. Biophys. Acta 512, 147.

MITCHELL G.F. & MILLER J.F.A.P. (1968) Cell to cell interaction in the immune response. II. The source of hemolysin-forming cells in irradiated mice given bone marrow and thymus or thoracic duct lymphocytes. J. Exp. Med. 128, 821.

PAPAHADJOPOULOS D., FRALEY R. & HEATH T. (1980) Optimization of liposomes as a carrier system for the intracellular delivery of drugs and macromolecules. In: Liposomes and Immunobiology, p. 151. (Ed. by B.H. Tom and H.R. Six). Elsevier/North Holland, New York.

PAPAHADJOPOULOS D., NIR S., OHKI S. (1972) Permeability properties of phospholipid membranes: effect of cholesterol and temperature. Biochim. Biophys. Acta 266, 561.

PAPAHADJOPOULOS D., VAIL W.J., JACOBSON K. & POSTE G. (1975) Cochleate lipid cylinders. Formation by fusion of unilamellar lipid vesicles. Biochim. Biophys. Acta 394, 483.

PATEL H.M. & RYMAN B.E. (1976) Oral administration of insulin by encapsulation within liposomes. FEBS Lett. 62, 60.

POSTE G., KIRSH R., RAZ A., SONE S., CORA B., FOGLER W.E. & FIDLER I.J. (1980) Activation of tumoricidal properties in macrophages by liposomes-encapsulated lymphokines: in vitro studies. In: Liposomes and Immunobiology, p. 93. (Ed. by B.H. Tom and H.R. Six). Elsevier/North Holland, New York.

RAHMAN Y.E., CERNY E.A., TOLLAKSEN S.L., WRIGHT B.J., NANCE S.L. & THOMSON J.F. (1974) Liposome-encapsulated actinomycin D: Potential in cancer chemotherapy. Proc. Soc. Exp. Biol. Med. 146, 1173.

RICHARDSON V.J., RYMAN B.E., JEWKES R.F., JEYASINGH K., TATTERSALL M.H.N., NEWLANDS E.S. & KAYE S.B. (1979). Tissue distribution and tumor localization of 99M-technetium labelled liposomes in cancer patients. Br. J. Cancer 40, 35.

RYMAN B.E., JEWKES R.F., JEYASINGH K., OSBORNE M.P., PATEL H.M., RICHARDSON V.J., TATTERSALL, M.H.N. & TYRRELL D.A. (1978) Potential applications of liposomes to therapy. Ann. N.Y. Acad. Sci. 308, 281.

RYMAN B.E. & TYRRELL D.A. (1980) Liposomes: Bags of potential. Essays Biochem. 16, 49.

SCHERPHOF G., DAMEN J. & HOEKSTRA D. (1981) Interactions of liposomes with plasma proteins and components of the immune system. In: Liposomes: From Physical Structure to Therapeutic Applications, p. 299. (Ed. by C.G. Knight). Elsevier/North Holland, New York.

SCHUSTER B.C., NEIDIG M., ALVING B.M. & ALVING C.R. (1979) Production of antibodies against phosphocholine, phosphatidylcholine, sphingomyelin, and lipid A by injecion of liposomes containing lipid A. J. Immunol. 122, 900.

SHAW I.H., KNIGHT C.G. & DINGLE J.T. (1976) Liposomal retention of a modified anti-inflammatory steroid. Biochem. J. 158, 473.

SHEK P.N. & LUKOVICH S. (1982) The role of macrophages in promoting the antibody response mediated by liposome-associated protein antigens. (Submitted for publication).

SHEK P.N. & SABISTON B.H. (1982a) Immune response mediated by liposome-associated protein antigens. I. Potentiation of the plaque-forming cell response. Immunology 45, 349.

SHEK P.N. & SABISTON B.H. (1982b) Immune response mediated by liposome-associated protein antigens. II. Comparison of the effectiveness of vesicle-entrapped and surface-associated antigens in immunopotentiation. Immunology (in press).

SIX H.R., KRAMP W.J. & KASEL J.A. (1980) Effects of liposomes on serological responses following immunization with adenovirus purified type 5 subunit vaccines. In: Liposomes and Immunobiology, p. 119. (Ed. by B.H. Tom and H.R. Six). Elsevier/North Holland, New York.

SUZUKI K. & TOMASI JR T.B. (1980) The regulatory effect of macrophages on the antigen-induced lymph node cell proliferative response. Cell. Immunol. 49, 317.

SZOKA F.C. & PAPAHADJOPOULOS D. (1980) Comparative properties and methods of preparation of lipid vesicles (liposomes). Ann. Rev. Biophys. Bioengin. 9, 467.

TAYLOR R.B. (1969) Cellular cooperation in the antibody response of mice to two serum albumins: specific function of thymus cells. Transplantn. Rev. 1, 114.

THOMSON A.W., FOWLER E.F. & PUGH-HUMPHREYS R.G.P. (1979) Immunopharmacology of the macrophage-toxic agent, carrageenan. Int. J. Immunopharmac. 1, 247.

TYRRELL D.A., HEATH T.D., COLLEY C.M. & RYMAN B. (1976) New aspects of liposomes. Biochim. Biophys. Acta 457, 259.

VAN HOUTE A.J., SNIPPE H. & WILLERS J.M.N. (1979) Characterization of immunogenic properties of haptenated liposomal model membranes in mice. I. Thymus independence of the antigen. Immunology 37, 505.

VAN HOUTE A.J., SNIPPE H., SCHMITZ M.G.J. & WILLERS J.M.N. (1981) Characterization of immunogenic properties of haptenated liposomal model membranes in mice. V. Effect of membrane composition on humoral and cellular immunogenicity. Immunology 44, 561.

VAN ROOIJEN N. & VAN NIEUWMEGEN R. (1977) Liposomes in immunology: the immune response against antigen-containing liposomes. Immunol. Commun. 6, 489.

VAN ROOIJEN N. & VAN NIEUWMEGEN R. (1980) Liposomes in immunology: evidence that their adjuvant effect results from surface exposition of the antigens. Cell. Immunol. 49, 402.

WEINBERGER O., HERRMANN S.H., MESCHER M.F., BENACERRAF B. & BURAKOFF S.J. (1980). Cellular interactions in the generation of cytolytic T lymphocyte responses: Role of Ia-positive splenic adherent cells in presentation of H-2 antigen. Proc. Natl. Acad. Sci. USA 77, 6091.

WEINBERGER O., HERRMANN S.H., MESCHER M.F., BENACERRAF B. & BURAKOFF S.J. (1981) Antigen-presenting cell function in induction of helper T cells for cytotoxic T-lymphocyte responses: Evidence for antigen processing. Proc. Natl. Acad. Sci. USA 78, 1796.

WEISSMANN G., KORCHAK H., FINKELSTEIN M., SMOLEN J. & HOFFSTEIN S. (1978) Uptake of enzyme-laden liposomes by animal cells in vitro and in vivo. Ann. N.Y. Acad. Sci. 308, 235.

WONG D.M. & HERSCOWITZ H.B. (1979) Immune activation by T-independent antigens: lack of effect of macrophage depletion on the immune response to TNP-LPS, PVP and dextran. Immunology 37, 765.

YASUDA T., DANCEY G.F. & KINSKY S.C. (1977) Immunogenicity of liposomal model membranes in mice: Dependence on phospholipid composition. Proc. Natl. Acad. Sci. USA 74, 1234.

YASUDA T., TADAKUMA T., PIERCE C.W. & KINSKY S.C. (1979) Primary in vitro immunogenicity of liposomal model membranes in mouse spleen cell cultures. J. Immunol. 123, 1535.

NUTRITIONAL CONSIDERATIONS IN IMMUNOTOXICOLOGY

D.F. Horrobin
Efamol Research Institute
P.O. Box 818, Kentville, Nova Scotia
Canada, B4N 4H8

If one attempts to use various information retrieval systems to find publications discussing the impact of nutrition on immunotoxicology, one comes up with nothing. There appears to be no literature which directly assesses this question. However, any immunotoxicological agent gaining access to a human or to an animal will be acting against a background of existing immunological function. Differences in background immunological status will therefore lead to differences in the actions of drugs. Background immunological status may be heavily dependent upon nutrition and in this sense nutrition is undoubtedly relevant to the assessment of the actions of immunotoxicological agents.

One interesting consequence of nutritional considerations is the choice of species to be used for investigations. The expression "guinea pig" rather than "rat" or "mouse" is the common lay word to describe humans involved in experimental situations. This is in spite of the fact that over the past thirty years guinea pigs have been used relatively rarely in animal studies in comparison to the rat and, especially in immunology, to the mouse. The common use of this term dates from the early days of this century when guinea pigs were the animals which were overwhelmingly important in medical research. They were important primarily because of all laboratory animals their responses to infections—and hence probably their immune status—were most close to those of humans. It is therefore interesting that, as will be discussed later, in two ways their nutritional metabolism is very similar to humans and quite different from that in mice and rats. Perhaps we should return to using guinea pigs as the major animal model if the main purpose of immunotoxicology is the investigation of the effects of toxic agents on human function.

The first part of the review will deal with the issue of malnutrition in general. The second will deal with a selected group of micronutrients which seem to have exceptionally important effects on immunological function.

NATO ASI Series, Vol. G2
Immunotoxicology. Edited by P. W. Mullen

MALNUTRITION

The close relationship between famine and epidemics is a commonplace which has been reported on innumerable occasions. Anyone who has travelled in less developed areas of the world carries back memories of children with infected eyes, noses and ears. It seems obvious that malnutrition leads to defective immunity with a greatly increased susceptibility to infection. Defining precisely the nature of that defect has, however, not proved easy. Many reports note that the worst infections appear to come not with famine, but with refeeding after the famine (Murray and Murray, 1977; McFarlane, 1976). Australian aboriginal children who were malnourished were resistant to viral infection (Jose, Welch and Doherty, 1970). Patients with anorexia nervosa, a psychiatric illness in which food intake is drastically reduced, are consistently resistant to viral infections. One of the factors which hinders their recovery is the rapid development of frequent infection once refeeding begins. This observation is not confined to humans. A diet low in protein given to mice may enhance rather than reduce their ability to reject skin grafts and may enhance _in vitro_ measures of cellular immunity (Good, Fernandes, Yunis, Cooper, Jose, Kramer and Hansen, 1976). Nevertheless, the overall effect of malnutrition, a situation in which there are deficiencies of the major food groups, together with deficiencies of many vitamins and minerals, is defective immune function. The whole subject has been reviewed in more detail by Chandra and Newberne (1977), McFarlane (1976) and Good _et al_ (1976).

Most of our knowledge about nutrition and immunity comes from the uncontrolled experiments of natural famine in which the precise nutritional deficiencies are unknown although obviously extensive. Many studies, the earliest dating from 1845 (McFarlane, 1976) have noted the severe atrophy of the thymus present in individuals dying from malnutrition. Later studies demonstrated that during starvation the thymus atrophies first, followed by the spleen, then the abdominal lymph nodes and then the cervical, axillary and popliteal nodes. In young children under the age of one, protein deficiency (kwashiorkor) seems to have the most severe effect, but beyond one both protein deficiency and total calorie deficiency (marasmus) seem equally damaging. Histological examination of the lymphoid organs in such children reveals almost total disappearance of lymphoid elements with replacement by fibrous tissue. Animal studies have led to similar observations but have shown that an apparently totally devastated thymus may be reconstituted within weeks by refeeding. Attempts to delineate more precisely the immunological defects in humans inevitably suffer from the conditions under which studies have to be carried out (McFarlane, 1976). Neutrophil leukocytes have reduced phagocytosis and chemotactic activity. T lymphocytes in vitro show reduced defences to both non-specific mitogens and to specific antigens whereas the B lymphocyte response to pokeweed mitogen is less suppressed. Matching the in vitro results are the depressed delayed hypersensitivity reactions to BCG vaccination or to DNCB injection, with normal or elevated levels of circulating IgG. Although total IgG levels are elevated, the responses to specific antigens such as vaccines, are often defective (McFarlane, 1976; Chandra and Newberne, 1977). This suggests that while overall IgG synthesis may be unimpaired, the production of specific antibodies which may require cooperation of T and B cells is impaired. Secretory IgA levels are consistently and unequivocally depressed, possibly accounting for the infections of ears, eyes, nose and throat and gastro-intestinal tract which are such features of malnutrition. One alarming observation which requires careful limitation of investigation is that in severely malnourished Australian aboriginal children, routine infant immunization procedures were followed by the deaths of as many as 50% of the immunized children (Kalokerinos, 1977). Similarly, smallpox vaccination in malnourished children may lead to generalized vaccinia (Vitteri, 1965). The additional stress seems to be too much for the severely defective responses.

It is obviously difficult to dissect out the precise mechanisms of immune failure in humans and some investigators have turned to animals to pursue their studies (McFarlane, 1976; Good et al, 1976). In general, human observations have been confirmed, that either protein or total calorie malnutrition will lead to atrophy of the thymus and lymphoid tissue. Beyond that the animal studies have been only modestly helpful and it seems doubtful how valid they are as guides to the human situation, partly because of the impossibility of imitating human famine and partly because of species differences. Chronic protein deficiency in mice enhanced graft versus host reactivity of spleen cells, enhanced allograft rejection and enhanced resistance to pseudorabies virus infection (Good et al, 1976), all manifestations of possibly enhanced T cell function. Total starvation, in contrast, severely depressed cellular immunity but enhanced humoral immunity. Rats with protein and calorie restricted diets were resistant to tumors (Good et al, 1976) apparently because of changes in the formation of blocking antibodies with reduction in all T cell function. In NZB/W mice, susceptible to development of autoimmune disease, a protein deficient diet enhanced both cellular and humoral immunity, delayed involution of the thymus but did not prolong life span. In contrast, the same strain of mice given a low calorie diet showed greatly extended life span. However, another short-lived strain of mice, DBA2, showed no extension of life span with a low calorie diet but did to a diet low in protein (Good et al, 1976). When there are such differences in responses of different strains of mice, one must have serious reservations as to the validity of animal experiments for human function.

Recently some doubt has been cast on the idea that the changes in the immune system are due to deficiency of any of the major nutrients. Golden, Golden, Harland and Jackson, (1978) have argued that any diet deficient in major food groups will also be deficient in zinc which, as will be discussed later, has profound effects on the immune system. In malnourished children he obtained remarkable growth of the thymus shadow on X-ray and in the skin response to DNCB by giving zinc alone. Similarly, Kalokerinos has noted that any form of malnourishment will lead to deficiency of vitamin C which also plays a key role in immunity. He drastically reduced deaths in aboriginal children due to immunization by administering vitamin C (Kalokerinos, 1977).

Regardless of the precise nutrients involved, there is evidence that enhanced adrenal corticosteroid secretion plays a key role in the atrophy of thymus and lymphoid tissue. Malnourished animals and humans have hypertrophied adrenals and elevated levels of glucocorticoids (McFarlane, 1976). Adrenalectomy in part prevents the thymus and lymphoid atrophy of malnutrition.

In concluding this section, it is obvious that malnutrition produces profound immunological abnormalities even though as yet we have little information about the precise mechanisms. It is also obvious that the actions of any immunotoxicological agents are likely to be dramatically greater in malnourished individuals. The effects of vaccination and immunization in such individuals provide awful warning of this.

OVERNUTRITION

There is much less evidence about the actions of excess nutrient intake on the immune system but there are some tantalizing clues. Diseases such as Crohn's disease and rheumatoid arthritis, which are generally believed to be auto-immune in nature, are much commoner in Western societies than in malnourished societies. Within Western societies, they appear to be much less common in vegetarians than in meat eaters (Lindahl, submitted for publication). McCay's experiments on rats showed that restriction of food intake could prolong life span. Walford (1980) has related this to the immune system. Walford has argued that the emergency of autoimmunity, in large part due to failure of T suppressor cell function, is a key determinant of aging. He has shown that dietary restriction, even if applied for the first time late in life, is able to inhibit the development of auto-antibodies and enhance T suppressor function. The inhibition of auto-immunity and prolongation of life in NZB/W mice given low calorie intakes (Good et al, 1976) points in the same direction. It is therefore clear that overnutrition as well as undernutrition has the potential for modulating the effects of immunotoxicants.

SPECIFIC ESSENTIAL NUTRIENTS

Specific nutrients may modulate the immunological function in at least three different ways:

(1) Because they are necessary for general metabolism, most essential nutrients are either co-factors for enzymes or constituents of enzymes. Many of these enzymes perform functions which are vital for all cells. If a deficiency of an essential nutrient is severe enough to disrupt metabolism in general, then inevitably the immune system will suffer. Severe deficiency of any essential nutrient will therefore lead to defective immune function (Scrimshaw, Taylor and Gordon, 1968).

(2) Because they are necessary for some specific aspect of metabolism which is vital for immune function. Some essential nutrients, while important generally, may also appear to have very specific effects on immunity. Vitamin C, zinc and essential fatty acids come into this category and will be discussed in greater detail later.

(3) Because they act as precursors for the formation of specific inflammatory mediators which play roles in the final common path of immunological responses. Histidine is a necessary precursor of histamine, tryptophan is a precursor of serotonin, essential fatty acids are precursors of prostaglandins, slow reacting substance of anaphylaxis (now identified as a leukotriene) and hydroxy acids, and tyrosine is a precursor of cathecholamines.

It is thus evident that deficiencies of highly specific essential nutrients may have profound effects on immunological status. The remainder of this section will be devoted to looking in greater detail at three of these nutrients: zinc, vitamin C, and essential fatty acids.

Zinc

Acrodermatitis enteropathica (AE) is a devastating inherited disease. Sufferers have no hair, little or no thymus, and severely defective immune function with susceptibility to many forms of infections including fungi which normally do little harm. They are effectively human "nude mice" although the parallel between the mouse and human syndromes has been largely ignored (Horrobin, Manku, Karmali, Morgan, Ally and Karmazyn, 1977).

In 1974 it was discovered that AE is a zinc deficiency disease, probably due to defective zinc absorption (Moynahan, 1977). Supplementation with high doses of zinc corrects all the abnormalities, stimulating hair growth and restoring normal immune function (Moynahan, 1977; Neldner and Hambidge, 1975). A similar disease in Friesian cattle responded similarly (Moynahan, 1974; Brummerstedt, Basse, Flagstad and Andresen, 1977). Zinc deficiency resulting from causes other than AE was also found to lead to profound immunodeficiency states with impairment of both humoral and cellular immunity (Srouji, Balisteri, Caleb, South and Starr, 1978). In normal humans with an unexplained low response of lymphocytes to PHA or con A, oral zinc sulphate significantly improved responsiveness (Duchateau, Delespesse and Vereecke, 1981). Similarly in patients with lymphoblastic leukaemia, zinc increased the number of rosette-forming cells (Wazewska-Czyzewska, Wesierska-Gadek and Lequtko, 1978). In humans with thymus atrophy and reduced delayed hypersensitivity reactions, zinc could restore thymus size and skin response.

Animal studies have confirmed the profound importance of zinc in immunological function. Zinc deficiency in rodents leads to dramatic atrophy of the thymus and impairment of both humoral and cellular immune responses, with marked drop in T cell, especially T helper cell, activity (Fraker Haas and Luecke, 1977; Fraker, DePasquale-Jardieu, Zwickl and Leuche, 1978; Gross and Newberne, 1980; Fernandes, Nair, Onoe, Tanaka, Floyd and Good, 1979; DePasquale-Jardieu and Fraker, 1979; Beach, Gershwin, Makishima and Hurley, 1980; Sandstead, 1973).

It therefore seems that zinc has some highly specific role to play in the thymus and lymphoid tissue and in T cell function. What that role is remains unknown. The similarities between the nude mouse and AE suggests that some critical metabolic step necessary for both hair and immune function is blocked. Since there is evidence that zinc deficiency is common in American and European populations, a test of any possible immunotoxicant in zinc deficient animals could be important as a guide to human use.

Vitamin C

Vitamin C, like zinc, is a nutrient which has many general roles in the body but which also seems to have some very specific function in the immune system. All the early reports of scurvy emphasize susceptibility to infection as a prominent feature (Lind, 1953; Bicknell and Prescott,

1953). Vitamin C levels are hign in the thymus, lymphocytes, neutrophils, macrophages and mast cells (Thomas and Holt, 1978). Lymphocytes seem to contain the highest vitamin C levels in the white cell fraction and unlike the situation with the neutrophils, the lymphocyte levels seem largely independent of the plasma concentrations, suggesting an active transport mechanism (Evans, Currie and Campbell, submitted for publication). There is a very strong inverse relationship between plasma ascorbic acid concentrations and histamine: when the ascorbic acid level was below 7mg/l, histamine levels rose sharply and ascorbic acid supplementation lowered them again (Clemetson, 1980). This suggests that vitamin C may control histamine release. There is good evidence that "normal" people may have low vitamin C levels especially in pregnancy (Moore, Rohatgi and Low, 1979).

Vitamin C seems to be essential for thymus growth (Dieter, 1971). Vitamin C deficient guinea pigs do not reject allografts (Kalden and Guthy, 1972) or develop experimental allergic encephalomyelitis (Meuller, Kies, Alvord and Show, 1962). In the former case parenteral vitamin C causes prompt graft rejection. In scorbutic guinea pigs levels of T lymphocytes were depressed and B lymphocytes enhanced (Fraser, Pavlovic, Kurahara, Murata, Peterson, Taylor and Feigen, 1980). Vitamin C supplementation restored normality over four weeks. In humans, oral vitamin C enhanced in vitro responsiveness to PHA (Delafuente and Panush, 1979). Also in humans, vitamin C deprivation led to an auto-immune disease similar to Sjogens's (Hood, Burns and Hodges, 1970).

Vitamin C also seems to have a particular role in regulating neutrophil function. In the Chediak-Higashi syndrome, neutrophils show defective chemotaxis and bacterial killing: vitamin C can correct these abnormalities (Boxer, Oliver, Allen and Baehner, 1976; Zurier, 1978). In patients with recurrent infections due to defective neutrophils, treatment with vitamin C alone normalized in vitro neutrophil function and prevented the infections (Rebora, Dallegri and Patrone, 1980).

There is also a great deal of evidence that vitamin C has an antimalignant effect (Cameron, Pauling and Leibovitz, 1979; Bram, Froussard, Gvichard, Jasmin, Augery, Sinoussi-Barre and Wray, 1980; Park, Amare, Savin and Hoogstraten, 1980). Whether this is related to its immunological actions remains to be determined.

The mechanism by which vitamin C enhances immune function is unknown. However, it does increase the formation of PGE_1, specifically (Horrobin, Oka and Manku, 1979). As the next section will demonstrate, PGE_1 may have a specific effect on T lymphocytes. The idea that PGE_1 is of particular importance in vitamin C action is enhanced by the finding that phenytoin, which produces a scurvy-like syndrome, can cause an auto-immune syndrome (Horrobin et al, 1979; Horrobin, 1980) just as can vitamin C deficiency (Hood et al, 1970).

Essential Fatty Acids (EFAs)

The effects of EFAs on the immune system are of exceptional interest because they operate on all the three levels mentioned at the beginning of this section.

(1) Essential fatty acids are essential constiuents of all cell membranes and are key determinants of membrane fluidity. They thus regulate functions of all cells and in view of the importance of membrane responses in the immune system are likely to have a key role.

(2) EFAs give rise to prostaglandins by the following reaction sequence:

Linoleic acid
↓
Gamma-linolenic acid
↓
Dihomogammalinolenic acid → 1 series PGs
↓
Arachidonic acid → 2 series PGs
Arachidonic acid → Leukotrienes

There are two types of PG derived from the main EFA, linoleic acid. 1 series PGs are formed from DGLA and PGE_1 seems to have a particular role in regulating thymus and T lymphocyte function. 2 series PGs are formed from arachidonic acid and may regulate both T lymphocytes and macrophages.

(3) Arachidonic acid is the source of a whole range of inflammatory mediators, including 2 series PGs, thromboxane A2, hydroxy acids and leukotrienes (the chemically defined major components of the slow reacting substance of anaphylaxis). PGs and thromboxane are formed by reaction sequences which start with the cyclo-oxygenase enzyme while the leukotrienes and hydroxy-acids are formed by a lipoxygenase enzyme sequence. Non-steroidal anti-inflammatory drugs such as aspirin and indomethacin block the cyclo-oxygenase while vitamin E blocks the lipoxygenase.

There is considerable evidence that PGE_1 is a key regulator of the thymus and of T lymphocytes. PGE_1 is found in large amounts in both animal and human thymus (Karim, Sandler and Williams, 1967; Horrobin, Manku and Oka et al, 1979). PGE_1 in vitro has actions similar to those of thymus hormone in causing maturation of T lymphocytes (Bach and Bach, 1974). Both zinc and vitamin C, which have thymic and T lymphocyte effects, are specific co-factors for the formation of PGE_1 (Horrobin et al, 1979). PGE_1 treatment of animals with adjuvant arthritis or of the NZB/W mouse prevents the development of the autoimmune disease, enhances T lymphocyte and depresses B lymphocyte function (Zurier and Quagliata, 1971; Zurier, Sayadoff, Torrey and Rothfield, 1977). Administration of evening primrose oil containing linoleic and gamma-linolenic acid, precursors of PGE_1, suppresses the development of adjuvant arthritis and experimental allergic encephalomyelitis (Kunkel, Ogawa, Ward and Zurier, 1981; Stackpoole and Mertin, 1981).

2 series PGs obviously play a substantial role in inflammation given the clinical inflammation reducing effects of NSAID. Leukotrienes also are involved and a full inflammatory response probably requires PGs, LTs and other mediators such as histamine and serotonin. Steroids block the release of arachidonic acid from membrane stores and so block the formation of both cyclo-oxygenase and lipoxygenase products. This may explain why they have greater clinical effectiveness than the NSAID.

In addition to their actions as inflammatory agents, there is also a good deal of evidence that PGs play a role as modulators of the immune response. The literature in this area is voluminous and bewildering. PGs are powerful agents which have biological actions over the range of 10^{-14} to 10^{-4} M. The in vivo concentrations at critical sites are unknown but what is known is that different concentrations of the same PG may have dramatically opposite effects (Horrobin, 1978; Horrobin, 1980). Most in vitro studies use only a single high concentration of a PG and therefore extrapolation from the in vitro to the in vivo situation is of uncertain value. What one can say is that the evidence is overwhelmingly in favor of an active role for 2 series PGs but the precise nature of that role is obscure. The subject has been well reviewed by Goodwin and Webb (1980). They point out that the main PG producing cell in human blood is probably the macrophage. Under some conditions, notably with sensitized cells, antibody production is enhanced by PGE_2 (Weider and Webb, 1981) but under most conditions 2 series PGs inhibit both T and B cell function. The immunosuppression of malignancy may be related to elevated production of PGs in this situation (Goodwin and Webb, 1980; Plescia, Smith and Grinwich, 1975). It is certain that our knowledge of

2 series PG effects is in its infancy and will have to be considerably developed before it makes much sense.

It is, however, clear that EFAs, for a whole variety of different reasons, are essential regulators of immune function. Recently it has become apparent that, although a simple linoleic acid deficiency in the diet is unlikely, many individuals may be functionally EFA deficient. This is because a variety of factors, including aging, alcohol, viral infections, diabetes, saturated fats and processed vegetable oils, can block the conversion of linoleic to gamma-linolenic acid (Horrobin, et al, 1979; Horrobin, 1980; Horrobin, 1981). This will lead to defects in formation of both 1 and 2 series PGs and is likely to have profound effects on immunological and inflammatory function. Particular interest therefore attaches to the idea of modifying immune function by by-passing the block by giving gamma-linolenic acid directly as evening primrose oil, or human milk, the only two substantial available sources.

Again investigation of immunological agents needs to take note of the fact that large parts of the population may have a functional EFA deficiency and studies should be done in animal models which to some degree imitate them.

OTHER CONSIDERATIONS: SPECIES AND DIET

One factor rarely considered in animal experiments is the type of protein fed. Little has been done on this in relation to immunology, but in the cardiovascular field different types of protein have dramatically different effects. Soy protein seems to protect against cardiovascular disease whereas casein exacerbates it (Horrobin, 1981). The effects of different proteins should therefore be checked as far as immunotoxicological studies are concerned.

The possibility of immunotoxicants having different effects in different species was alluded to earlier. Two of the reactions which seem critically important in the metabolism of nutrients which play key immunological roles, show major species differences. In both cases the guinea pig and human are similar and are quite different from rats and mice.

(1) Dependence on dietary vitamin C. Rats and mice make their own Vitamin C and greatly increase its production rate in response to any form of stress. Guinea pigs and humans require dietary vitamin C and cannot respond to stress as do rats and mice.

(2) Activity of the delta-5-desaturase, the enzyme which converts DGLA to arachidonic acid. In adult rats and mice this enzyme is highly active, leading to ready formation of arachidonic acid from dietary

linoleic acid. In humans and guinea pigs this enzyme has little activity, leading to the idea that much of the arachidonic acid available for synthesis of leukotrienes and 2 series PGs must come from the diet. Most of the dietary arachidonic acid comes from meat which could explain why vegetarians seem resistent to inflammatory disease.

Guinea pigs have long been known to have immune systems which in some ways are more similar to humans than are those of rats and mice. These two metabolic steps may be part of the explanation.

CONCLUSION

It is clear that nutrients may have profound effects on immunological function and also that nutrient intakes in the population are widely variable. Assessments of immunotoxicants must take into consideration the fact that, among others, many humans in any population are likely to have suboptimal intakes of zinc, vitamin C and essential fatty acids. Animal studies must therefore be designed with these factors in mind.

REFERENCES

BACH, M.A. and BACH, J.F. (1974) Effects of prostaglandins and indomethacin on rosette forming lymphocytes: interactions with thymic hormone. Prostaglandin Synthetase Inhibitors (HJ Robinson and JR Vane, eds), Raven Press, NY, 241.

BEACH, R.S., GERSHWIN, M.E. MAKISHIMA, R.K. and HURLEY, L.S. (1980) Impaired immunologic autogeny in postnatal zinc deprivation. J. Nutr. 110, 805.

BICKNELL, F. and PRESCOTT, F. (1953) The Vitamins in Medicine. Grune and Stratten, New York.

BOXER, L.A., OLIVER, J.M., ALLEN, J.M., BAEHNER, R.L. (1976) Improvement in vitro of polymorphonuclear leucocyte function in the Chediak-Higashi syndrome by ascorbic acid and A23187. Blood 48, 988.

BRAM, S., FROUSSARD, P., GUICHARD, M., JASMIN, C., AUGERY, Y., SINOUSSI-BARRE, F. and WRAY, W. (1980) Vitamin C preferential toxicity for malignant melanoma cells. Nature 284, 629.

BRUMMERSTEDT, E., BASSE, A., FLAGSTAD, T. and ANDRESEN, E. (1977) Animal model of human disease. Acrodermatitis enterpathica, zinc malabsorption. Am J.Pathol. 87, 725.

CAMERON, E., PAULING, L. and LEIBOVITZ, B. (1979) Ascorbic acid and cancer: a review. Cancer Res. 39, 663.

CHANDRA, R.K. and NEWBERNE, P.M. (1977) Nutrition, Immunity and Infection. Plenum Press, New York.

CLEMETSON, C.A.B. (1980) Histamine and ascorbic acid in human blood. J.Nutr. 110, 662.

DELAFUENTE, J.C. and PANUSH, R.S. (1979) Augmentation of human lymphocyte responses by vitamin C. Clin. Res. 27, 323A.

DEPASQUALE-JARDIEU, P. and FRAKER, P.J. (1979) The role of corticosterone in the loss in immune function in the zinc deficient A/J mouse. J. Nutr. 109, 1847.

DIETER, M.P. (1971) Further studies on the relationship between vitamin C and thymic humoral factor. Proc. Soc. Exp. Biol. Med, 136, 316.

DUCHATEAU, J., DELESPESSE, G. and VEREECKE, P. (1981) Influence of oral zinc supplementation on the lymphocyte response to mitogens of normal subjects. Am. J. Clin. Nutr. 34, 88.

EVANS, R.M., CURRIE, L. and CAMPBELL, A. (submitted for publication) The distribution of ascorbic acid between various cellular components of blood in normal individuals and its relation to the plasma concentration.

FERNANDES, G., NAIR, M., ONOE, K., TANAKA, T., FLOYD, R. and GOOD, R.A. (1979) Impairment of all-mediated immunity functions by dietary zinc deficiency in mice. Proc. Nat. Acad. Sci. USA 76, 457.

FRAKER, R.J., DEPASQUALE-JARDIEU, P., ZWICKL, C.M. and LEUCHE, R.W. (1978) Regeneration of T cell helper function in zinc-deficient adult mice. Proc. Nat. Acad. Sci. USA 75, 5660.

FRAKER, P.J., HAAS, S.M. and LUECKE, R.W. (1977) Effect on zinc deficiency on the immune response of the young adult A/J mouse. J. Nutr. 107, 1889.

FRASER, R.C., PAVLOVIC, S., KURAHARA, C.G. MURATA, A., PETERSON, N.S., TAYLOR, K.B. and FEIGEN, G.A. (1980) The effect of variations in vitamin C intake on the cellular immune response of guinea pigs. Am J. Clin. Nutr. 33, 839.

GOLDEN, M.H.N., GOLDEN, B., HARLAND, P.S.E.G. and JACKSON, A.A. (1978) Zinc and immunocompetence in protein-energy malnutrition. Lancet 2, 1226.

GOOD, R.A., FERNANDES, G., YUNIS, E.J., COOPER, W.C., JOSE, D.C., KRAMER, T.R. and HANSEN, M.A. (1976) Nutritional deficiency, immunologic function and disease. Am. J. Pathol. 84, 599.

GOODWIN, J.S. and WEBB, D.R. (1980) Regulation of the immune response by prostaglandins. Clin. Immunol. Immunopath. 15, 106.

GROSS, R.L. and NEWBERNE, P.M. (1980) The role of nutrition in immunologic function. Physiol. Rev. 60, 188.

HOOD, J., BURNS, C.A. and HODGES, R.E. (1970) Sjogren's syndrome in scurvy. New Eng. J. Med. 282, 1120.

HORROBIN, D.F. (1978) Prostaglandins: Physiology, Pharmacology and Clinical Significance. Eden Press, Montreal.

HORROBIN, D.F. (1980) Regulation of prostaglandin biosynthesis: negative feedback mechanisms and the selective control of formation of 1 and 2 series prostaglandins: relevance to inflammation and immunity. Med. Hypothesis 6, 687.

HORROBIN, D.F. (1981) Loss of delta-6-desaturase as a key factor in aging. Med Hypotheses 7, 1211.

HORROBIN, D.F. The regulation of prostaglandin biosynthesis by the manipulation of essential fatty acid metabolism. Rev. Pure. Appl. Pharmacol. Sci,, in press.

HORROBIN, D.F., MANKU, M.S., KARMALI, R.A., MORGAN, R.P., ALLY, A.I. and KARMAZYN, M. (1977) Immunological deficiency, cancer and prostaglandins. Br. Med. J. 2, 1086.

HORROBIN, D.F., MANKU, M.S. and OKA, M. et al (1979) The nutritional regulation of T lymphocyte function. Med. Hypotheses 5, 969.

HORROBIN, D.F., OKA, M. and MANKU, M.S. (1979) The regulation of prostaglandin E1 formation: a candidate for one of the fundamental mechanisms involved in the actions of vitamin C. Med. Hypotheses 5, 849.

JOSE, D.G., WELCH, J.S. and DOHERTY, R.L. (1970) Humoral and cellular immune responses to streptococci, influenza and other antigens in Australian aboriginal school children. Australian Paed. J. 6, 192.

KALDEN, J.R. and GUTHY, E.A. (1972) Prolonged skin allograft survival in vitamin C deficient guinea pigs. Bur. Surg. Res. 4, 114.

KALOKERINOS, A. (1977) Every Second Child. Aboriginal Medical Service. Sydney, Australia.

KARIM, S.M.M., SANDLER, M. and WILLIAMS, E.D. (1967) Distribution of prostaglandins in human tissues. Br. J. Pharmacol. 31, 340.

KUNKEL, S.L., OGAWA, H., WARD, P.A. and ZURIER, R.B. (1981) Suppression of chronic inflammation by evening primrose oil. Progress in Lipid Research, 20, 885.

LIND, J. (1953) A Treatise of the Scurvy, 1753. Sands, Murray and Cochran, Edinburgh. Reprinted, Edinburgh University Press.

LINDAHL, O. (submitted for publication) Fasting and a vegetarian diet in treatment of rheumatoid arthritis.

McFARLANE, H. (1976) Malnutrition and immunity. In Immunological Aspects of Foods (N. Catsinpoolas, ed). Air Publishing Co., Westport, pp. 372-387.

MEULLER, P.S., KIES, M.W., ALVORD, E.C., and SHOW, G.M. (1962) Prevention of experimental allergic encephalomyelitis by vitamin C deprivation. J. Med. 115, 329.

MOORE, M.R., ROHATGI, S. and LOW, R.A.L. (1979) Prenatal and postnatal maternal leucocyte ascorbic acid concentrations. Br. J. Olstet. Gynae. 86, 293.

MURRAY, M.J. and MURRAY, A.B. (1977) Starvation suppression and refeeding activation of infection, an ecological necessity? Lancet 1, 123.

MOYNAHAN, E.J. (1974) Acrodermatitis enterpathica: a lethal inherited human zinc deficiency disorder. Lancet 2, 399.

MOYNAHAN, E.J. (1977) Zinc deficiency and cellular immunodeficiency in acrodermatitis enteropathica in man and zinc deficiency with thymus hypoplasia in Friesian calves: a possible genetic link. Lancet, 2, 1057.

NELDER, K.H. and HAMBIDGE, K.M. (1975) Zinc therapy of acrodermatitis enteropathica. New Eng. J. Med. 292, 879.

PARK, C.H., AMARE, M., SAVIN, M.A. and HOOGSTRATEN, B. (1980) Growth suppression of human leukemic cells in vitro by L-ascorbic acid. Cancer Res. 40, 1062.

PLESCIA, O.J., SMITH, A.H. and GRINWICH, K. (1975) Subversion of the immune system by tumor cells and role of prostaglandins. Proc. Nat. Acad. Sci. USA, 72, 1848.

REBORA, A., DALLEGRI, F. and PATRONE, F. (1980) Neutrophil dysfunction and repeated infections: influence of levamisole and ascorbic acid. Br. J. Derm. 102, 49.

SANDSTEAD, H.H. (1973) Zinc nutrition in the United States. Am. J. Clin. Nutr. 26, 1251.

SCRIMSHAW, N.S., TAYLOR, C.E. and GORDON, J.E. (1968) Interactions of nutrition and infection. World Health Organization, Geneva.

SROUJI, M.N., BALISTERI, W.F., CALEB, M.H., SOUTH, M.A. and STARR, S. (1978) Zinc deficiency during parenteral nutrition: skin manifestations and immune incompetence in a premature infant. J. Pediat. Surg. 13, 570.

STACKPOOLE, A. and MERTIN, J. (1981) The effect of prostaglandin precursors in in vivo models of cell mediated immunity. Progress in Lipid Research 20, 649.

THOMAS, W.R. and HOLT, P.G. (1970) Vitamin C and Immunity: an assessment of the evidence. Clin. Bcp. Immunol. 32, 370.

VITTERI, F. cited by BROWN, R.E. and KATZ, M. (1965) Antigenic stimulation in malnourished children. East Afr. Med. J. 42, 221.

WALFORD, R. (1980) Immunology and aging. Am. J. Clin. Path. 74, 247.

WAZEWSKA-CZYZEWSKA, M., WESIERSKA-GADEK, J. and LEGUTKO, L. (1978) Immunostimulatory effect of zinc in patients with auto lymphoblastic leukaemia. Folia. Haematol. 105, 727.

WEIDER, K.J. and WEBB, D.R. (1981) The effect of prostaglandin metabolism on immunoglobulin and antibody production in naive and educated whole spleen cells. Prostaglandins Med. 7, 79.

ZURIER, R.B. (1978) Prostaglandins and cyclic neucleotides in the Chediak-Higashi syndrome and experimental systemic lupus erythematosus. J. Invest. Dermatol. 71(1), 36.

ZURIER, R.B., SAYADOFF, D.M., TORREY, S.B. and ROTHFIELD, N.F. (1977) Prostaglandin E treatment in NZB/NZW mice. Arthritis Rheum. 20, 723.

ZURIER, R.B. and QUAGLIATA, F. (1971) Effect of prostaglandin E1 on adjuvant arthritis. Nature 234, 304.

RISK-BENEFIT ASSESSMENT IN IMMUNOTOXICOLOGY

Helen Tryphonas, M.Sc. and Ian C. Munro, Ph.D.
Toxicology Research Division, Bureau of Chemical Safety
Food Directorate, Health Protection Branch
Health and Welfare, Tunney's Pasture
Ottawa, Ontario, Canada, K1A 0L2

The potentially harmful effects of chemicals on the immune system of laboratory animals and inadvertently on the health of man are being increasingly recognized at the regulatory and consumer levels. Immunotoxicity of a varying degree has been produced in experimental animals by certain environmental contaminants, numerous chemicals that may enter the food chain at the manufacturers levels, and chemicals used intentionally for therapeutic purposes (Vos, 1977). Exposure to these chemicals is practically unavoidable, while the use of others serves a genuinely beneficial purpose in food processing. Furthermore, a wide variety of chemicals used in medicine have been shown to confer overwhelming benefits to mankind. Yet, inherent in the use of or exposure to, many of these chemicals is the element of risk to the human population. The process of risk assessment is being recognized as essential to every organized human society. Consequently, the delicate balancing of health and other benefits against the "perceived" risks has become the central issue in the development of regulatory policy (Munro and Krewski, 1981).

Regulatory decisions regarding the establishment of safe levels of potentially toxic chemicals require a careful evaluation of many factors, including health, economic and social parameters. Ultimately, the risk-analysis process will involve the selection among viable options that are physically and biologically realizable. Quite often, however, decisions must be made at a time when not all facts concerning the effects of chemicals on health are available and one must not take any risks in waiting for the generation of such data. In view of the importance attached to regulatory decisions, regulatory agencies are actively engaged in the quest for additional parameters of improved sensitivity over those existing which can be used in evaluating toxicological insults of potentially harmful chemicals. One such area of investigation is immunotoxicology, the subdiscipline of immunology which is concerned with detrimental immune modulation by chemicals. The applicability of immunotoxicology to the overall toxicological assessment of a chemical is based on the presumption that immune responses are very sensitive and alterations of this system can be expected at levels which may not show other

NATO ASI Series, Vol. G2
Immunotoxicology. Edited by P. W. Mullen

observable health effects. The immune response involves a large network of organs and a variety of cell types that carry out interrelated functions. Responsiveness to external challenges is governed by a complex regulatory network of highly specialized cellular populations and subpopulations intricately connected through numerous avenues of communications (Bier, Dias da Silva, Goetze and Mota, 1981).

Chemicals are known to affect the immune system and ultimately its several functions ar various levels of the immunologic tree. They may affect the afferent limb of the immune response, which influences monocyte/macrophage numbers and function, B-cell number and function or T-cell number and function at the level of antigen uptake, processing and presentation to lymphocytes or they may affect the central portion of the immune response. Modulation of the latter portion of the immune response would be affected by agents which modify either or both: 1) cellular DNA synthesis and, 2) function of suppressor cells, helper cells and effector B and T cells. Lastly, the effect of chemicals could be on the efferent portion of the immune response which expresses the immune effector functions developed during the central portion of the response (Braun and Harris, 1981). Ultimately, any immunosuppressive effects induced by chemicals will result in one or more of the following: 1) reduced ability of the animal to combat infection, 2) changes in the immune surveillance mechanism resulting in increased number and incidence of tumors, 3) development of hypersensitivity in susceptible individuals and 4) the initiation of certain changes in host-related antigens which may eventually lead to autoimmune diseases. It is in the context of these main areas that immunotoxicity can be of potential usefulness in assessing the level of risk associated with a particular chemical.

According to the World Health Organization (1961) <u>risk</u> is defined as "the likelihood of suffering a harmful effect or effects resulting from exposure to a risk factor (usually some chemical or physical or biological agent). Risk is usually expressed as the probability of occurrence of an adverse effect, i.e. the expected ratio between the number of individuals that would experience an adverse effect in a given time and the total number of individuals exposed to the risk factors". An in-depth analysis of this definition will reveal that the process of risk assessment, and its evaluation in relationship to the benefits derived from the use of a chemical, is a multi-dimensional process requiring certain basic prerequisites which we usually do not have in immunotoxicology. Firstly, one needs to obtain a qualitative, and most importantly, a numerical estimate, of the individual components of the "perceived" risk and benefits. Secondly, it is equally important to know the level of significance assigned to each component, and thirdly, one needs to estimate the relative importance of these various components. It becomes apparent, therefore, that the risk-benefit analysis in immunotoxicology is a large and awkward problem.

The difficulties encountered in this type of analysis are partly due to our incomplete understanding of the complex regulatory mechanisms that govern interactions within the immune system, and partly due to the deficiencies in the type of immunological data available. The latter can be attributed to the fact that immunotoxicology is a relatively new area of investigation. Consequently, the sensitivity of methods employed in assessing immunotoxicity and the significance of results when extrapolated to man, are under continuous scrutiny similar to that observed for carcinogenicity and mutagenicity testing. Therefore, during these initial stages of immunotoxicology, efforts are being made to develop and standardize a tier of immunological functional assays with suitable degrees of sensitivity and high levels of reproducibility to facilitate data comparison among the various laboratories. To fulfill this objective, investigators have experimented with chemicals, usually at high doses, in in vivo and in vitro tests and many of these have produced valuable data indicating that some chemicals may alter the immune system and its many functions in a manner which can be detrimental to the health of man (Vos, 1977). This information is undoubtedly useful in arriving at a conclusion regarding the qualitative aspect of the effect, but it is lacking in information needed to quantitatively assess the risk involved in each case.

For example, we are all familiar with the tremendous benefits derived from the use of pesticides. It has been estimated that approximately 20-30 per cent of food would be spoiled world-wide due to insect infestation, molds or other diseases, if it were not for the use of chemicals (World Health Organization, 1961). Such an action contributes indirectly to the general health of the individual by providing better quality and safer nutrition. However, in recent years evidence has been accumulated to indicate that certain pesticides may affect the immune system of animals and inadvertently the health status of man (Vos, 1977; Sharma and Zeeman, 1980). It is therefore, the magnitude of the risk that needs to be calculated in light of the known benefits derived from the use of these chemicals. Data available on one such chemical, namely, DDT, will be considered to illustrate the difficulties encountered in any attempt to quantitate this risk. Experimental results pertaining to the effect of DDT on antibody production to several antigens in seven species including the goldfish, chicken, duck, rat, guinea pig, rabbit and humans have been compiled by Sharma and Zeeman (1980).

Depending on several factors, i.e. the species studied, the dose and regimen of DDT administration, and the antigen employed, one may see no effect, or increases in antibody production, or even an initial increase followed by a depression in the secondary phase of antibody production. It is also apparent that the outcome of antigenic challenge would be influenced by the schedule of testing, i.e. the interval between antigen challenge and study of the effect, or the time of administration of the chemical, i.e. whether it was given before, after, or simultaneously with, the antigen.

Even if one considers results from different immunotoxicologic assays presumably measuring different functions or responses, one finds that the threshold level at which immunotoxicity can be detected varies with any given chemical. For example, in the experiment by Street and Sharma (1975), an attempt was made to establish dose-response relationships for DDT, Aroclor 1254, Carbaryl, and Methylparathion by feeding a series of clinically subtoxic amounts of these pesticides to rabbits. A number of functional parameters were measured including; the antibody response to sheep erythrocytes (SRBC), quantitation of serum globulin levels, skin sensitivity to tuberculin and enumeration of lymph node antibody producing cells. Immunosuppression was detected at the lowest dosage level (0.03 mg/kg/day) as indicated by reduced numbers of antibody producing cells in lymph nodes, numbers of germinal centers in the spleen, or the status of the thymus cortex, but effects were appreciable only at the highest treatment dose when evaluating skin sensitivity to tuberculin. Quantitation of serum g-globulin showed an intermediate threshold level while specific antibody formation against SRBC was not affected.

Conflicting results of this nature are by no means restricted to DDT studies alone. Similar studies on the effects of other chemicals have also given incoherent results. The compound 2,3,7,8-tetrachlorodibenzo-p-dioxin (TCDD) (a highly toxic impurity that may be formed during the production of 2,4,5-trichlorophenol), di-n-octyltin-dichloride (DOTC) and di-n-butyltin-dichloride (DBTC), have also shown to be immunosuppressive in certain species while no effect was detected when a different species was used. But even if we ignore the interspecies differences and we accept the effect, for example, on mouse thymus atrophy as being directly mediated by the chemical in question, one finds it difficult to comprehend the biological significance of this effect in terms of human health and consequently evaluate the level of risk involved. This is further complicated when one finds only negligible effects of the same chemical on the ability of lymphocytes to transform in the presence of PHA, or no effect on the susceptibility of the same species of animal to pseudorabies infection (Vos, 1977; Gupta, Vos, Moore, Zinkl and Bullock, 1973; Seinen and Willems, 1976).

Similarly, incomplete results have been produced by other environmental contaminants including the metals of lead, mercury and the widely studied polychlorinated biphenyl compounds (PCBs). Although these chemicals have been shown to be immunosuppressive in a variety of functional tests (Street and Sharma, 1975; Loose, Pittman, Benitz and Silkworth, 1977; Loose, Silkworth, Pittman, Benitz and Mueller, 1978; Thomas and Hinsdill, 1978; Koller and Brauner, 1977), others have reported either no effect or an effect in selected tests or species only (Lawrence, 1980; Gaworski and Sharma, 1978).

Accordingly, extrapolation to man of the observed immunosuppressive effects of chemical in animals and the evaluation of the possible risks becomes very difficult. This task is further complicated by the observed species specificity and individual susceptibility to immunotoxicants. For example, thymus atropy has been observed to be caused by TCDD in all species studied, but the effects of the chemicals, DBTC and DOTC are shown to be species (rat) specific. In this respect the superior value of data produced in primates and man whenever possible is undisputable. After all, it is the potentially harmful effects on man continuously exposed to small amounts of chemicals that is of primary concern. Consequently, the data showing a severe effect of DBTC and DOTC on human in vitro thymocyte transformation by PHA and ConA mitogens, would be more revealing with respect to the risk involved than the slight effect produced by the same chemical on rat lymphocytes upon being transformed by the same mitogens (Vos, 1977). In interpreting these results one must also keep in mind that the immune system of the host offers several pathways for handling a challenge. Consequently, a component of the pathway may be compromised by a toxic insult, yet the host's ability to survive a challenge by an infectious agent may be unchanged. However, since the primary objective is to minimize risk, one should be concerned for compromises of any component of the immune system even though the host's ability to survive infection may seem to be unchanged.

Undoubtedly, epidemiological studies of humans exposed to these chemicals and follow-up studies would yield information useful in evaluating the risk size. Such information would indicate whether the effects on the immune system are short-lived and therefore of negligible significance or the damage is permanent in which case, the risk to man from infection or cancer could reach potentially unacceptable levels. One must be aware, however, of the limitations of these studies, since the variability resulting from human social behaviour, the time scale involved, and the changes imposed on our environment when adverse effects are suspected can modify the results of any epidemiological study.

In addition to environmental contaminants, a variety of other chemicals used for therapeutic purposes are known to modify the immune response at different levels giving rise to a broad spectrum of reactions similar to those discussed earlier (Braun and Harris, 1981; Sterzl, 1980). Consequently, the benefits derived from the use of any drug must always be weighed against possible risks. The risk-benefit equation will fluctuate depending on the condition to be treated. For example, in the case of self-limiting minor ailments, the benefits must always significantly outweigh the risks. However, in rare diseases, where the prognosis is poor and no other effective therapy exists, it is probably justifiable to take great risks, but always with a consideration of the hazards of remaining untreated. For example, the risks involved in using chemicals which are immunosuppressive and anti-inflammatory in certain situations as in, for example, the chemotherapy of some forms of cancer, may be far outweighed by the hazards of remaining untreated.

However, many of these chemicals are being widely used, and often for long terms, as immunosuppressive and anti-inflammatory agents in patients with non-neoplastic conditions affecting the connective (rheumatoid arthritis, systemic lupus erythematosus, scleroderma, dermatomysitis); renal (nephrotic syndrome, glomerulonephritis, transplant rejection); gastrointestinal (ulcerative colitis, granulomatous colitis, chronic active hepatitis); neurologic (multiple schlerosis, myasthenia gravis); hematologic (autoimmune hemolytic anemia, idiopathic thrombocytopenic purpura, erythrocyte aplasia) and dermatologic (psoriasis, pemphigus) tissues (Schein and Winokur, 1975). In addition, patients with specific types of malignancies have gained in recent years substantial increases in survival as a result of improvements in cancer chemotherapy. All these groups of patients are at risk for the development of long-term complications resulting from treatment. It is in these groups of patients that the process of evaluation of the risks becomes difficult since the effects on the immune system may not be manifested clinically until the damage has become severe and irreversible.

For example, one of the alkylating agents, cyclophosphamide has been used in the control of a variety of experimentally produced inflammatory disease states, and in malignant and autoimmune conditions in man. Cyclophosphamide has been shown to produce in appropriate doses and schedules, a decrease in macrophage number and function in guinea pig and human peripheral blood, and, at levels of 300mg/kg, has also been shown to deplete lymphocytes from B-dependent areas in lymph nodes, spleen and bone marrow in many species without substantially affecting lymphocytes in the T-dependent areas of these tissues. These effects, however, have proven to be reversible in short-term exposure experiments. Consequently, the risk to humans, in cases where its use is deemed necessary, can be reduced by manipulating the dose and period of exposure to the chemical (Finch, 1980). In addition to its short-term use, however, cyclophosphamide has been applied extensively in the treatment of systemic lupus erythematosus (SLE) and is claimed to reduce the dose of steroids required for treatment. Evidence has been accumulated to show that such long-term exposure to cyclophosphamide leads to the formation of bladder tumors resulting in death or requiring drastic surgery (Elliott, Essenhigh and Morley, 1982). Cyclophosphamide has also been used along with other immunosuppressive drugs for the purpose of preventing rejection of kidney transplants. Kinlen et al. have estimated an excess frequency of malignancy, mainly from malignant lymphoma and skin tumors occurring during the first four years after immunosuppressive treatments. These treatments carried a 1.3 per cent risk of tumor induction and a 0.4 per cent risk of mortality from the induced tumors during the period of observation (Kinlen, Sheil, Peto and Doll, 1979). Can an acceptable level of risk be calculated for the use of cyclophosphamide? It is obvious that in order to justly assess the level of acceptable risk one needs to look at the survival rate of SLE patients not receiving the cyclophosphamide treatment or the problems and hazards resulting from renal dialysis.

In addition to these chemicals, many of the antimicrobial agents are known to be immunosuppressive under certain circumstances (Finch, 1980). The risk to man as a result of the immunosuppressive effect of these agents is probably very small since antimicrobial chemotherapy is usually of short duration and the effects reversible. However, the magnitude of the risk becomes important in cases of protracted use of antimicrobial chemotherapy in chemoprophylaxis of rheumatic fever and recurrent urinary tract infections, in the treatment of tuberculosis, leprosy, deep seated bone infection, systemic mycoses and acne vulgaris (Finch, 1980). Immune mechanisms play an integral part in the pathogenesis of several of these conditions and are also important for recovery. These infections are frequently opportunistic and may often occur in patients already immunocompromised by virtue of underlying malignant disease or as a result of antimitotic and immunosuppressive therapy. Consequently, close monitoring of patients receiving antimicrobial chemotherapy is of paramount importance.

In summary the process of risk-benefit assessment in immunotoxicology is a large, multidimensional process which seeks to measure the probability and severity of unwanted and adverse immune modulation(s) produced by low levels of chemicals in man. The determined levels of risk to man for any given chemical will fluctuate depending on the frequency with which new evidence for its toxic effects becomes available.

Although benefits derived from the use of a chemical can often be recognized and enumerated with a high level of precision, a qualitative and particularly a quantitative assessment of its risks based on available immunotoxicological data, is not possible at present. This is particularly true of pesticides and other environmental contaminants for which our knowledge of their mechanism of action is poor and the available animal data are often incomplete or, at best, inconclusive. Considerable variation is noted in nearly all known factors involved in risk assessment. There is great variation in risk between chemicals, due to their individual physico-chemical properties, the amounts used and the length of exposure. The effect of exposure will vary with dose, the route of administration, the ability of an animal to repair damage, and the specific detoxification mechanisms and pharmacokinetic characteristics observed. Assessment of risk is further complicated by the realization that chemicals behave differently not only in different species, but often among different strains of the same species, the latter being dependent upon individual sensitivity.

Presently, the primary concern of immunotoxicity studies is the development in animals of a battery of in vivo and in vitro assays which can be used as sensitive indicators of exposure to, or the effects of, a chemical at dose levels comparable with those to which the human population is actually being exposed. Such animal experimentation may be useful as a means of defining the appropriate immune parameters meriting consideration when investigating a compound's potential immunotoxicity in man. The ultimate value of any data derived from animal studies in determining the degree to which a risk is considered acceptable under a given set of circumstances, however, will depend upon the qualitative and quantitative accuracy of its extrapolation to man. This degree of accuracy is usually indicated from the outcome of carefully designed epidemiological studies conducted on populations exposed to the chemical(s) for long periods of time or from "post-marketing surveillance data" in the case of drugs. It is only through a cautious and in-depth analysis of all available data that a relatively acceptable level of risk can be estimated for any particular chemical. Such data should be derived from well designed and executed studies in a variety of laboratory animals. A battery of in vivo and in vitro assays with the appropriate sensitivity and reproducibility must be employed and the most sensitive indicators of toxicity should be determined for each chemical considered. Functional tests on the immune system of humans (exposed and non-exposed to the chemical of concern) must also be performed whenever possible.

As a final caveat in designing such experiments one must bear in mind that a wide variety of environmental, physiological, and pathological conditions can also influence the immune system. In particular, the hormones of the adeno-hypophysis may exert a direct or indirect effect on the structure and function of the lymphoid organs and on the phagocytic activity of macrophages. Other factors including the potential immuno-regulatory effect of α-fetoprotein and malnutrition should also be taken into consideration when conducting immunotoxicity tests (Vos, 1977).

REFERENCES

BIER, O.G., DIAS DA SILVA, W., GOETZE, D., MOTA, I. (1981) Fundamentals of Immunology. Springer-Verlag, New York

BRAUN, D.P. and HARRIS, J.E. (1981) Modulation of the immune response by chemotherapy. Pharmac. Ther. 14, 89.

ELLIOTT, R.W., ESSENHIGH, D.M. and MORLEY, A.R. (1982) Cyclophosphamide treatment of systemic lupus erythematosus: Risk of bladder cancer exceeds benefit. Brit. Med. J. 284, 1160.

FINCH, R. (1980) Immunomodulating effects of antimicrobial agents. J. Antimicrob. Chemoth. 6, 691.

GAWORSKI, C.L. and SHARMA, R.P. (1978) The effects of heavy metals on [^{3}H]-thymidine uptake in lymphocytes. Toxicol. Appl. Pharmacol. 46, 305.

GUPTA, B.N., VOS, J.G., MOORE, J.A., ZINKL, J.G. and BULLOCK, B.C. (1973) Pathologic effects of 2,3,7,8-tetracholordibenzo-p-dioxin in laboratory animals. Environ. Health Perspect. 5, 125.

KINLEN, L.J., SHEIL, A.G.R., PETO, J. and DOLL, R. (1979) Collaborative United Kingdom-Australasian study of cancer in patients treated with immunosuppressive drugs. Br. Med. J. 2, 1461.

KOLLER, L.D. and BRAUNER, J.A. (1977) Decreased B-lymphocyte response after exposure to lead and cadmium. Toxicol. Appl. Pharmacol. 42, 621.

LAWRENCE, D.A. (1980) Metal mediated modulation of B-cell proliferation and differentiation. Federation Proc. 39, 917.

LOOSE, L.D., PITTMAN, K.A., BENITZ, K.F. and SILKWORTH, J.B. (1977) Polychlorinated biphenyl and hexachlorobenzene induced humoral immuno-suppression. J. Reticuloendothel. Soc. 22, 253.

LOOSE, L.D., SILKWORTH, J.B., PITTMAN, K.A., BENITZ, K.F. and MUELLER, W. (1978) Impaired host resistance to endotoxin and malaria in poly-chlorinated biphenyl and hexachlorobenzene treated mice. Infect. Immunity 20, 30.

MUNRO, I.C. and KREWSKI, D.R. (1981) Risk assessment and regulatory decision making. Fd. Cosmet. Toxicol. 19, 549.

SCHEIN, P.S. and WINOKUR, S.H. (1975) Immunosuppressive and cytotoxic chemotherapy: Long-term complications. Ann. Inter. Med. 82, 84.

SEINEN, W. and WILLEMS, M. (1976) Toxicity of orgonotin compounds. I. Atrophy of thymus and thymus dependent lymphoid tissue in rats fed di-n-octyltindichloride. Toxicol. Appl. Pharmacol. 35, 63.

SHARMA, R.P. and ZEEMAN, M.G. (1980) Immunologic alterations by environmental chemicals: Relevance of studying mechanisms versus effects. J. Immunophar. 2(3), 285.

STERZL, J. (1980) Immunopharmacology and its toxicological problems. Arch. Toxicol. Suppl. 4, 109.

STREET, J.C. and SHARMA, R.P. (1975) Alteration of induced cellular and humoral immune responses by pesticides and chemicals of environmental concern: Quantitative studies of immunosuppression by DDT, aroclor 1254, carbaryl, carbofuran, and methylparathion. Toxicol. Appl, Pharmacol. 32, 587.

THOMAS, P.T. and HINSDILL, R.D. (1978) Effect of polychlorinated biphenyls on the immune responses of rhesus monkeys and mice. Toxicol. Pharmacol. 44, 41.

VOS, J.C. (1977) Immune suppression as related to toxicology, CRC Critical Reviews in Toxicology. May 1977, 67-101.

WORLD HEALTH ORGANIZATION (1961) Principles coverning consumer safety in relation to pesticide residues. Technical Report No. 240, WHO. Geneva.

IMMUNOTOXICOLOGY: THE VIEWPOINT OF AN INDUSTRIAL IMMUNOLOGIST

G.E. Davies
Imperial Chemical Industries PLC
Central Toxicology Laboratory
Alderley Park Nr Macclesfield
Cheshire SK10 4TJ, England

A number of untoward consequences can result from a disordered immune response and it is therefore appropriate that we should consider such disorders which arise from exposure to drugs and other chemicals, i.e. to immunotoxic compounds. Immunotoxicology could be defined as: 'the undesirable effects of an inappropriate response of the immune system'; 'inappropriate' in that many of the 'undesirable effects' might in other circumstances be both desirable and appropriate, for instance a heightened antibody response is desirable for certain protective effects against infection but undesirable in some cases of auto-immunity.

A number of schemes, many of which will be described at the present meeting, have been devised for the purpose of examining new chemicals for immunotoxicity, and a major aim of these tests must be to identify immunotoxic compounds on a prospective, predictive basis. In practice some of the compounds selected for intensive study have been chosen because of evidence suggesting that human exposure had in fact deviated the immune response. Such parallel observations in man and animals would at first sign appear to offer an ideal situation for assessing the validity of animal models.

The use of existing chemicals and the introduction of new ones is quite properly controlled by governmental regulatory agencies. So far, apart from tests for contact allergy, regulations have not yet appeared for 'immunotoxic compounds'. As an immunologist employed by a chemical company, I am naturally concerned about the current state of the subject, about the strategy and tactics of the use of animal models currently in vogue and about possible future developments in the legislative field. Let me at once declare that I am not intending to use any argument to lessen the efforts we should make towards safer compounds but I would like to share with you some of the doubts that have occurred to me in surveying the present scene.

My main approach has been to examine the literature on some of the more studied 'immunotoxic' compounds, paying particular attention to the

NATO ASI Series, Vol. G2
Immunotoxicology. Edited by P. W. Mullen

(sometimes contradictory) effects reported in man, and then to compare these with the effects reported in animals. In this way I hoped to be able to consider how predictive the animal tests would have been had they preceded human exposure. I have also considered two other situations met with in practice; the problems associated with idiosyncratic reactions, which by definition occur in a majority of the exposed populations and are frequently unpredictable, and then those untoward events in man which are labelled 'immunological' but for which such an attribution seems to be without a proven basis.

ANIMAL TESTS

If tests for toxicity in animals are to have any useful predictive value and this, surely, is a major objective, then there are a number of considerations that they must take into account. These are:

Reproducibility
Species, strain, age and sex of animals
Dose-response
Endocrine influence
Diurnal and seasonal variation

Many of these points have been dealt with in an excellent paper by Sharma and Zeeman (1980) and I need to do little more than re-emphasize some of their cogent observations.

Reproducibility in the present context does not mean simply the ability to obtain the same answer by repeating the same observation (this is largely a matter of technical competence in experimental design and performance) but it also includes the ability to arrive at the same answer by differing approaches. Sharma and Zeeman (1980) tabulate some results published on DDT which, according to the conditions of testing, may have either no effect, or increase, or decrease antibody formation, and they list some of the reasons for these disparate results: dose, and dosing schedule; nature of antigen; interval between antigen challenge and effects studied. Many other sources of variability are quoted in the literature and it is sufficient to mention only a few illustrative examples. Verschuuren, Ruitenberg, Peetcoom, Helleman and van Esch (1970) found that triphenyltin acetate was more immunosuppressive in guinea pigs than in rats and that females were more affected than males. The effect of age on the immune response is well-known. Vos (1980) has emphasised that animals may be particularly susceptible during ontogeny. Compounds may depress the production of one class of immunoglobulin and stimulate another: Speirs, Takenaka, Benson and Jones (1980) showed that cyclophosphamide could suppress the IgM and IgG response but stimulate IgE production depending on the timing of administration. Sharma and Zeeman (1980) have commented on the lack of dose-response studies and in this connection it is worthwhile considering the relationship between the dose which is immunotoxic in animals and the amount consumed by man: Spreafico, Vecchi, Mantovani, Tagliabue, Sironi, Luini and Garattini (1981) for example, calculated that a 60Kg man would need to consume more than 130mg of saccharin to excrete the same amount of saccharin in urine as did rats minimally immunosuppressed with the chemical. Seasonal (Godfrey, 1975) and circadian (Pownall, Kabler and Knapp, 1979) rhythms can profoundly affect the immune response and endocrine (particularly adrenocortical) influences are well recognized.

STUDIES IN MAN

As was pointed out in my introduction, some of the chemicals studied for immunotoxic effects in animals were selected because there appeared to be evidence of immunotoxicity in man. I have chosen three such compounds and have reviewed briefly the nature and extent of the human evidence, and then referred to the, sometimes discordant, results of the animal tests.

Polybrominated Biphenyls (PBB)

Attention was drawn to these compounds when Bekesi, Holland, Anderson, Fishbein, Rom, Wolff and Selikoff (1978) reported functional abnormalities in the peripheral blood of Michigan dairy farmers who comsumed food accidentally contaminated with the material. Subsequent studies by this group (Bekesi, Roboz, Anderson, Roboz, Fishbein, Sellikoff and Holland (1979) showed that the abnormalities included decreased numbers of T-cells, an increase in lymphocytes with no detectable surface markers and a decreased response of the peripheral lymphocytes to mitogens *in vitro*. The significance of these findings has been questioned by Silva, Kauffman, Simon, Landrigan, Humphrey, Heath, Wilcox, Van Amburg, Kaslow, Ringel and Hoff (1979) who found no differences in the numbers or functions of various classes of lymphocytes in high - or low PBB exposure or control groups and they suggested that "Bekesi's positive findings are artifactual". It is noteworthy that Bekesi's group (Bekesi *et al*, 1979) themselves were unable to detect a consistent correlation between delayed cutaneous hypersensitivity responses and impaired lymphocyte function. Of possibly greater importance is the finding in a major study (Barr, 1980) of no significant immunological difference between exposed and control children. Meester (1979) examined a group of farmers exposed to PBB: 55% complained of loss of energy and easy fatiguability; 38% joint pain; 31% headaches; 24% muscle pain; 20% dizziness; 19% backaches; 19% joint stiffness; 17% blurry vision; 17% somnolence; 16% nervousness; 15% skin rashes; 17% abdominal complaints; 11% irritability and 10% diarrhoea. Such findings, although obviously not related to an immune response, illustrate the difficulty of human studies.

An interesting hypothesis to explain altered response of lymphocytes to mitogen stimulation was proposed by Howard, Werner and Sleight (1980). They showed that sows exposed to PBB had increased blood levels of very low density lipoproteins which, they suggest, could reflect an altered lipid metabolism related to the hepatotoxicity of PBB which in turn altered the lipid composition of lymphocyte membranes and hence their response to mitogens.

Brown and Jones (1981) reported on 2567 workers exposed to the related polychlorinated biphenyls (and for those compounds also there is animal evidence of immunotoxicity). The mortality from all causes as well as the cancer mortality was lower in the exposed group (apart from a statistically non-significant increase in rectal and liver cancer).

In contrast to this confusing situation in man, animal studies are in agreement that polyhalogenated biphenyls are immunosuppressive; but if we applied the concepts enunciated so clearly by Sharma and Zeeman (1980), might we not, conceivably, have demonstrated the opposite effects?

TCDD

The compound which has received the greatest attention in animal tests on immunotoxicity is probably 2,3,7,8-tetrachlorodibenzo-p-dioxin (TCDD) - and on a dose-basis it is certainly the most potent (Dean, Luster, Boorman, Chae, Lauer, Luebke, Lawson and Wilson, 1981) and yet an official study of the 'Seveso' incident where a large population had been exposed accidentally to TCDD, found no significant difference in immune function between exposed and control children (Seveso, 1979). Indeed a 20 month follow-up study claimed that "on account of the small TCDD exposure the population has had no severe damage by this accident". It is of course possible that a more detailed examination or a longer-term study might reveal untoward effects but they are not yet apparent.

Cimetidine

This drug is a competitive antagonist of histamine H_2 receptors and is used clinically for the control of gastric acid secretion. The presence of the H_2 receptors on lymphocytes (Plaut, Lichtenstein, Gillespie and Henney, 1973) gave presumptive evidence that cimetidine could modulate the immune response and indeed a number of published reports suggest that it might do so. Smith, Couhig, Miller and Salaman (1979), Robertson, Peden, Saunders, Gibbs, Pott, Brown, Wormsley and Beck (1979) and Palacios and Alarcon-Segovia (1981) found that lymphocytes from patients dosed with cimetidine had an enhanced response to phytomitogens in vitro; Gifford, Schmidlke and Ferguson (1981) found a similar enhancement of the mixed lymphocyte response, and Avella, Madsen, Bindor and Askenase (1978) demonstrated an increased delayed-hypersensitivity skin test. In contrast McGregor, Cochran, Ogg, Smith, Gillespie and Forrestor (1977), De Pauw, Lamers, Wagener and Festen (1977) and Festen, De Pauw and Wagener (1981) were unable to demonstrate an immunological abnormality in patients dosed with cimetidine.

Animal experiments are sparse. Smith et al (1979) and Festen, Berden and Koene (1980) were unable to show any effect of cimetidine on the homograft reaction in rodents. Lipsmeyer (1980) found that administration of cimetidine to guinea pigs increased MIF production in vitro but had no effect on delayed hypersensitivity skin tests.

These three examples serve to illustrate my contention that the current series of tests in animals do not inevitably predict the likely outcome in man and such a state of affairs is, to me at least, confusing.

IDIOSYNCRACY

It is a characteristic of toxic effects that they are dose-related; given a large enough dose all the population will respond. However, many undesirable effects of drugs and other chemicals frequently are seen in only a small proportion of an exposed population (the classical example is allergy but this aspect of the problem is not dealt with here).

It is unlikely that animal tests will ever be able to predict the appearance of such reactions. Their very rarity suggests a multi-factorial cause, one example being genetic predisposition. On occasion selection of the correct strain of animals can be helpful. For instance the production of auto-immune glomerulonephritis by mercury is seen only in the Brown Norway rat, but observations of this nature depend to a large extent on serendipity, leading to the discovery of a susceptible strain. In instances such as this the immunologist is probably well advised to reserve his expertise for a post hoc investigation.

PSEUDO-IMMUNE SYNDROMES

I have applied this term to those untoward events in man which are reputed to be immunological but the evidence at best is circumstantial, and occasionally even the result of an imprecise technique. I have chosen two examples of which I have personal experience, and for each example I have indicated the relevance of animal tests.

Halothane

Anaesthesia with halothane is followed, on rare occasions, by a severe hepatitis. The true incidence of this undesirable side-effect is difficult to establish - a figure of about 1 : 10,000 is usually quoted but a group at the London Hospital (Strunin and Simpson, 1972) showed that only a small proportion of these are 'unexplained hepatitis following halothane' - and most of them follow multiple exposures. Several hypotheses, none yet fully substantiated, have been proposed to explain this phenomenon (I have elsewhere discussed the improbability that it is an allergic response (Davies and Holmes, 1972 and Davies, 1973)) but immunosuppression is the explanation most commonly offered by anaesthetists. It has been suggested that the condition is in fact a viral hepatitis, previously kept in check by an immune response and allowed to become manifest by the immunosuppression which accompanies anaesthesia (Johnstone, 1964).

Numerous studies in animals and man have shown that anaesthesia - per se, not necessarily associated with an anaesthetic - is accompanied by a profound, although transient, immunosuppression. Now I am not here concerned with the correctness or otherwise of this explanation of the cause of the hepatitis but it would seem difficult to establish a link between generalised, non-specific immunosuppressive effects of anaesthetics in animals and a response to a particular anaesthetic with an incidence of 1 in 10,000.

Vinyl Chloride

Lange, Juhe, Stein and Veltman (1974) introduced the term 'vinyl chloride-induced disease' for a multi-system disorder which included dysfunction of the liver and lungs, splenomegaly, osteolysis, sclerodermatous skin changes and thrombocytopenia in some workers engaged in the production of polyvinyl chloride. Ward, Udnoon, Watkins, Walker and Darke (1976) suggested that vinyl chloride (VC) disease was an 'immune-complex' disorder. The presence of immune complexes was not demonstrated directly but was inferred from the findings of mixed cryoglobulins, *in vivo* conversion of complement and depressed values of C4 and C3. Cryoglobulins associated with Raynaud's phenomonon due to VC were also detected by Langauer-Lewowicka, Dudziak, Byczkowska and Marks (1976). Ward and colleagues (1976) also claimed that there was a reduction in the T-cell population, but their evidence for this is unconvincing. They suggested that reactive metabolites of vinyl chloride might act as haptens (although no evidence for relevant antibodies was sought) or that a metabolite produced a conformational change in IgG molecules. Animal tests, so far, have not been helpful in elucidating the problem. The activity of murine lymphocytes *in vitro* was either increased (Sharma and Gehring, 1979) or unaffected (Thurman, Simms, Goldstein and Kilian, 1978). No effect was seen in rabbits (Sharma, Yakel and Gehring, 1980) but delayed hypersensitivity was depressed in guinea pigs (Hicks and Sahyoun, 1980). None of this work in animals revealed the presence of immune complexes.

GENERAL CONSIDERATIONS

Where does all this leave me? I must confess to a vague feeling of unease. Toxicity testing in general is concerned with the relationship between Hazard and Risk. Hazard can be defined as what could happen, and Risk as what is likely to happen. Animal experiments can play a valuable role in the definition of Hazard — even though, as with DDT, apparently opposite effects are demonstrable. Such studies did however reveal conditions where such opposite effects could occur.

Risk assessment is much more complex and depends on a multitude of considerations, including risk/benefit ratios (how essential is the compound?), size of exposed population, level and period of exposure, nature of hazard, etc. Animal experiments, therefore, provide some of the terms in the complex equation describing risk, but they cannot be the whole equation.

A separate, but equally cogent consideration is the cost-effectiveness of testing. It can be argued that no cost is too great to ensure the safety of the public and this argument is unanswerable. But it can be asserted with equal cogency that a point may be reached where the cost of ensuring such safety is so great as to make manufacture of the product in question uneconomic. I have an uneasy feeling that some of the more elaborate schemes for immunotoxicity testing are on the verge of pricing themselves out.

Rather more frivolous comments would include my perception that immunotoxicology appears to hold the record for the ratio of the number of review articles to original papers, and the perception of the dominance of a small number of research centres — the names of Dean and Vos occur with astonishing frequency in any bibliographic list. I hope, however, that they will both accept this comment in the spirit in which it is offered, namely one of admiration — and envy!

CONCLUSIONS

My criticisms of some of the published studies in humans must not be taken to imply that immunotoxicity cannot occur in man: this would be a patent absurdity. Similarly, my comments about the predictive value of animal tests may simply reflect the bewilderment which results from a study of the literature. We must seriously consider the role of the immunologist in toxicological studies: should he devote his attention primarily to the design of screening tests or should emphasis be placed on events occurring in man (i.e. a 'trouble-shooting role')? In my experience compounds with a specific immunotoxic effect are rarely seen — in the course of testing several thousand new compounds, over many years, in the search for immunomodulatory drugs, no such specific effect was found whereas I have been involved in two major studies resulting from untoward events in man (viz. practolol and halothane).

A major conclusion of this paper is that there is a discordance between published studies of immunotoxic effects in man and in animals. It seems to me important that industrial and academic scientists, of different scientific disciplines (immunologists, pharmacologists, biochemists, chemists, pathologists, etc) should collaborate in an organized fashion to further research in this area. It is my firmly-held opinion that such collaborative effort is required before regulatory requirements are imposed.

REFERENCES

AVELLA, J., MADSEN, J.E., BINDER, H.J. and ASKENASE, P.W. (1978) Effect of histamine H_2-receptor antagonist on delayed hypersensitivity. Lancet 1, 624.

BARR, M. (1980) Pediatric aspects of the Michigan polybrominated biphenyl contamination. Envir. Res. 21, 255.

BEKESI, J.G., HOLLAND, J.F., ANDERSON, A.J., FISHBEIN, A.S., ROM, W., WOLFF, M.S. and SELIKOFF, I.J. (1978) Lymphocyte function of

Michigan dairy farmers exposed to polybrominated biphenyls. Science 199, 1207.

BEKESI, J.G., ROBOZ, J., ANDERSON, H.A., ROBOZ, J.P., FISHBEIN, A.S., SELLIKOFF, I.J. and HOLLAND, J.F. (1979) Impaired immune function and identification of polybrominated biphenyls (PBB) in blood compartments of exposed Michigan dairy farmers and chemical workers. Drug & Chem. Toxicol. 2, 179.

BROWN, D.P. and JONES, M. (1981) Mortality and industrial hygiene study of workers exposed to polychlorinated biphenyls. Arch. Envir. Hlth. 36, 120.

DAVIES, G.E. (1973) Is halothane hepatotoxicity an allergic reaction to halothane? Proc. Roy. Soc. Med. 66, 55.

DAVIES, G.E. and HOLMES, J.E. (1972) Drug-induced immunological effects on the liver. Brit. J. Anaesth. 44, 941.

DEAN, J.H., LUSTER, M.I., BOORMAN, G.A., CHAE, K., LAUER, L.D., LUEBKE, R.W., LAWSON, L.D. and WILSON, R.E. (1981) Assessment of immunotoxicity induced by the environmental chemicals 2,3,7,8-tetrachlorodibenzo-p-dioxin, diethylstilbestrol & benzo/a/pyrene. p. 37. In: Advances in Immunopharmacology. (eds. Hadden, J., Chedid, L., Mullen, P. and Spreafico, F.) Pergamon Press, Oxford.

FESTEN, H.P.M., BERDEN, J.H.M. and KOENE, R.A.P. (1980) Cimetidine does not acceletate skin graft rejection in mice. Clin. Exp. Immunol. 40, 193.

FESTEN, H.P.M., DePAUW, B.E., SMEULDERS, J. and WAGENER, D.J.T. (1981) Cimetidine does not influence immunological parameters in man. Clin. Immunol. Immunopathol. 21, 33.

GIFFORD, R.R.M., SCHMIDTKE, J.R. and FERGUSON, R.M. (1981) Cimetidine modulation of lymphocytes from renal allograft recipients. Trans. Proc. 13, 663.

GODFREY, H.P. (1975) Seasonal variation of induction of contact sensitivity and of lymph node T lymphocytes in guinea pigs. Int. Arch. Allergy App. Immunol. 49, 411.

HICKS, R. and SAHYOUN, H.A. (1980) Immunosuppressive effects of vinyl chloride monomer on delayed hypersensitivity in the guinea pig. Brit. J. Pharmacol. Proc. 10-12 Sept., 553.

HOWARD, S.K., WERNER, P.R. and SLEIGHT, S.D. (1980) Polybrominated biphenyl toxicosis in swine: effects on some aspects of the immune system in lactating sows and their offspring. Toxicol. Appl. Pharmacol. 55, 146.

JOHNSTONE, M. (1964) Liver injury in the surgical patient: a critical review. Brit. J. Anaesth. 36, 718.

LANGE, C-E., JUHE, S., STEIN, G. and VELTMAN, G. (1974) Die sogenannte vinyl chlorid-krank-heit-eine berufsbedingte systemsklerose? Int. Arch. Arbeitsmed. 32, 1.

LANGAUER-LEWOWICKA, H., DUDZIAK, Z., BYCZKOWSKA, Z. and MARKS, J. (1976) Cryoglobulinemia in Raynaud's Phenomenon due to vinyl chloride. Int. Arch. Occup. Envir. Hlth. 36, 197.

LIPSMEYER, E.A. (1980) Effect if cimetidine on delayed hypersensitivity. Immunopathology 16, 166.

McGREGOR, C.J.A., COCHRAN, A.J., OGG, L.J., SMITH, I.S., GILLESPIE, G. and FORRESTOR, J. (1977) Immunological and other laboratory studies of patients receiving short-term cimetidine therapy. Lancet 1, 122.

MEESTER, W.D. (1979) The effect of polybrominated biphenyls on man: the Michigan PBB disaster. Vet. Hum. Toxicol. 21, Suppl. 31, 5.

PALACIOS, R. and ALARCON-SEGOVIA, D. (1981) Cimetidine abrogates suppressor T cell function in vitro. Immunol. Letters 3, 33.

DePAUW, B.E., LAMERS, C.B.H.W., WAGENER, D.J.T. and FESTEN, H.P.M. (1977) Immunological studies after long-term H_2-receptor-antagonist therapy. Lancet 2 , 616.

PLAUT, M., LICHTENSTEIN, L.M., GILLESPIE, E. and HENNEY, C.S. (1973) Studies on the mechanism of lymphocyte mediated cytolysis. IV. Specificity of the histamine receptor on effector T-cells. J. Immunol. 111, 389.

POWNALL, R., KABLER, P.A. and KNAPP, M.S. (1979) The time of day antigen encounter influences the magnitude of the immune response. Clin. Exp. Immunol. 36, 347.

ROBERTSON, A.J., PEDEN, N.R., SAUNDERS, J.H.B., GIBBS, J.H., POTTS, R.C., BROWN, R.A., WORMSLEY, K.G. and BECK, J.S. (1979) Cimetidine and the immune response. Lancet 2 , 420.

SEVESO (1979) The escape of toxic substances at the ICMESA establishment on 10th July 1976 and the consequent dangers to health and the environment due to industrial activity. A translation by the Health and Safety Executive of the official report of the Parliamentary Commission of Enquiry, by permission of the Parliament of the Republic of Italy.

SHARMA, R.P. and GEHRING, P.J. (1979) Immunologic effects of vinyl chloride in mice. Ann. N.Y. Acad. Sci. 320, 551.

SHARMA, R.P., YAKEL, H.O. and GEHRING, P.J. (1980) Immunotoxicologic studies with vinyl chloride in rabbits and mice. Int. J. Immunopharmac. 2, 295.

SHARMA, R.P. and ZEEMAN, M.G. (1980) Immunologic alterations by environmental chemicals: relevance of studying mechanisms versus effects. J. Immunopharmacol. 2, 285.

SILVA, J., KAUFFMAN, C.A., SIMON, D.G., LANDRIGAN, P.J., HUMPHREY, H.E.B., HEATH, C.W., WILCOX, K.R., Van AMBURG, G., KASLOW, R.A., RINGEL, A. and HOFF, K. (1979) Lymphocyte function in humans exposed to polybrominated biphenyls. J. Reticuloendothel. Soc. 26, 341.

SMITH, M.D., COUHIG, E., MILLER, J.J. and SALAMAN, J.R. (1979) Cimetidine and the immune response. Lancet 1, 1406.

SPEIRS, R.S., TAKENAKA, T., BENSON, R.W. and JONES, J.M. (1980) Models for assessing the effects of toxicants on immunocompetence of mice. III. Augmentation by IgE antibody response to tetanus toxoid by cyclophosphamide in mice. J. Envir. Pathol. Toxicol. 4, 383.

SPREAFICO, F., VECCHI, A., MANTOVANI, A., TAGLIABUE, A., SIRONI, M., LUINI, W. and GARATTINI, S. (1981) The assessment of the immunotoxicity of xenobiotics: experience with tetrachlorodibenzdioxin and saccharin. p. 295. In: Advances in Immunopharmacology. (eds. Hadden, J., Chedid, L., Mullen, P. and Spreafico, F.) Pergamon Press, Oxford.

STRUNIN, L. and SIMPSON, B.R. (1972) Halothane in Britain today. Brit. J. Anaesth. 44, 919.

WARD, A.M., UDNOON, S., WATKINS, J., WALKER, A.E. and DARKE, C.S. (1976) Immunological mechanisms in the pathogenesis of vinyl chloride disease. Brit. Med. J. 1, 936.